Beyond the Drill

A STRATEGIC GUIDE FOR DENTISTS ON LAUNCHING AND LEADING A DENTAL STARTUP

Hussam Asker, DDS

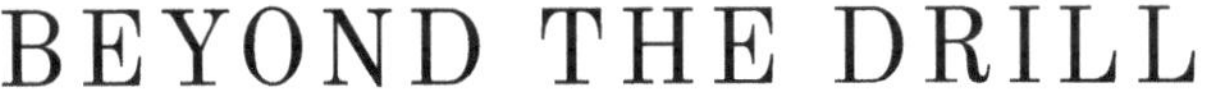
BEYOND THE DRILL

Contents

Disclaimer

The information contained in this book is for general informational purposes only. The author makes no representations or warranties of any kind, express or implied, about the completeness, accuracy, reliability, suitability, or availability of the information contained herein. Any reliance you place on such information is therefore strictly at your own risk. In no event will the author be liable for any loss or damage including without limitation, indirect or consequential loss or damage, or any loss or damage whatsoever arising from loss of data or profits arising out of, or in connection with, the use of this book. This book offers no financial, legal, or any professional or dental advice. It is meant for educational purposes only for dentists and dental students. Through this book, you are able to link to other websites that are not under the control of the author. The author has no control over the nature, content, and availability of those sites. The inclusion of any links does not necessarily imply a recommendation or endorse the views expressed within them. Every effort is made to keep the book up and running smoothly. However, the author takes no responsibility for, and will not be liable for, the book being temporarily unavailable due to technical issues beyond our control. The views and opinions expressed in this book are those of the author and do not necessarily reflect the official policy or position of any other agency, organization, employer, or company. The mention of specific companies or products within the book does not imply a recommendation or endorsement by the author unless explicitly stated. All content provided in this book is for informational purposes only. The author makes no representations as to the accuracy or completeness of any information in this book. The author will not be liable for any errors or omissions in this information nor for the availability of this information. The author will not be liable for any losses, injuries, or damages from the display or use of this information. The information contained in this book is derived from the author's comprehensive self-education efforts, including listening to podcasts, conducting online research, reading academic literature, and leveraging professional experiences. These experiences notably include serving as an associate dentist and successfully leading a dental startup project.

I

Introduction

1. Overview of Entrepreneurial Dentistry

Growing up in a small town in Lebanon, where access to dental care was once scarce, I witnessed firsthand the transformative power of a single dentist with a vision. My father, a pioneer in our community, established one of the first dental practices in his town, laying the foundation for a family legacy built on entrepreneurship and patient care. Witnessing his dedication sparked a fire within me, igniting a passion for both dentistry and the entrepreneurial spirit it inherently held.

From Lebanon to Ann Arbor, Michigan: Chasing the American Dream and the Future of Dentistry

Fueled by this passion, I ventured to the United States, pursuing my education at the prestigious University of Michigan School of Dentistry. While honing my clinical skills, I began to understand the pivotal role entrepreneurship plays in shaping the future of dentistry. It wasn't just about treating teeth; it was about building practices, making patient-centered decisions, and navigating the ever-evolving healthcare landscape.

Dentistry at a Crossroads: Technology, Transformation, and the Human Touch

The landscape of dentistry is undergoing a seismic shift. Technological advancements and artificial intelligence are both challenging and amplifying the entrepreneurial spirit. The traditional "small business" model faces threats from commoditization, potentially sacrificing the personalized touch that defines our profession.

A Call to Action: Embracing the Entrepreneurial Spirit

This book delves into the core concepts of entrepreneurship in dentistry, and the pivotal role you, as a new dentist, play in shaping its future. Through personal anecdotes and professional insights, I aim to inspire you to embrace entrepreneurship not just as a career path, but as a way to uphold the values that make dentistry a noble and impactful field.

Your Journey Begins Now: Stepping into Your Leadership Role

Graduation isn't the end; it's the beginning of your entrepreneurial journey. You are not just a dentist; you are a potential leader poised to shape the future of dental care. The dental entrepreneurship path offers autonomy, innovation, and the ability to build a practice that reflects your values and vision.

Beyond Financial Freedom: Reclaiming the Essence of Dentistry

Choosing entrepreneurship isn't just about financial independence; it's about reclaiming the essence of dentistry as a *small business.* It's about resisting the commoditization of your profession and safeguarding the patient-centered approach that defines it. **You are a specialized professional, not a cog in a machine**. Your skills, experience, and commitment set you apart.

Embrace the Challenge, Lead with Confidence

Embracing entrepreneurship is a call to reclaim control of your professional destiny. It's a call to lead with confidence, leveraging your intelligence, leadership skills, and determination to carve your own path. See this not just as a path to financial success, but as a way to safeguard the integrity and individuality of your chosen profession.

Navigating the Entrepreneurial Path vs. the DSO Expedition

Owning a dental office is akin to embarking on a thrilling entrepreneurial adventure, where every decision carries weight and every milestone achieved is a testament to your vision and hard work. However, the journey of building a dental practice shares striking similarities with the broader world of business, particularly in the choices one faces at the outset.

Picture this: you're at a crossroads, contemplating how to bring your dental dreams to life. You can take the path of the pioneer, meticulously crafting a business plan, devising operational systems, and painstakingly building your practice from the ground up. This route demands creativity, resilience, and an unwavering belief in your ability to turn your vision into reality.

On the other hand, there's the allure of the franchise model—a well-trodden path where the blueprints for success have already been drawn. Instead of reinventing the wheel, you can align yourself with a proven system, tapping into their established support networks. It's like having a roadmap to success handed to you on a silver platter, allowing you to focus on executing the plan rather than conceptualizing it from scratch.

Enter the Dental Support Organization (DSO), the franchise model's dental counterpart. As a DSO-affiliated dentist, you're essentially stepping into the shoes of a **franchisee**, while the DSO serves as the **franchisor**, providing you with a ready-made playbook for practice management. These DSOs have honed their systems through years of experience across various dental practices, offering a turnkey solution for dentists looking to hit the ground running.

But here's where things get interesting: while the franchise model may seem like a shortcut to success, it comes with its own set of caveats. Unlike traditional business franchises with ironclad contracts and stringent guidelines, the dental franchise landscape operates within a more nebulous regulatory framework. This means that while DSOs may not have you sign on the dotted line, their influence over your practice can be just as pervasive.

Imagine being handed a playbook with unwritten rules—expectations subtly implied rather than explicitly stated. From the types of insurance you accept to the protocols you follow, every aspect of your practice is subject to the guiding hand of the DSO. While some DSOs may tout their commitment to ethical standards and dentist autonomy, the bottom line often reigns supreme, leading to pressures to conform to established norms for the sake of profitability.

Nevertheless, the allure of the DSO model persists for many dentists, particularly those who crave structure and support in their practice management endeavors. For them, the idea of relinquishing some autonomy in exchange for a proven system and a built-in support network is a small price to pay for peace of mind and financial security.

In the end, whether you choose the entrepreneurial route or opt for the safety net of a DSO, the journey of owning a dental practice is a thrilling ride filled with challenges, triumphs, and everything in between. It's a testament to the resilience and ingenuity of dentists everywhere as they navigate the ever-evolving landscape of modern dentistry.

Join me on this exciting journey: In the coming chapters, we'll delve into the practical aspects of opening and managing a dental practice, empowering you with the knowledge and guidance to turn your entrepreneurial dream into a reality. Remember, you have the capacity to be both a dentist and a business owner, a combination that ensures both professional fulfillment and exceptional patient care.

2. Beyond Graduation: Charting Your Dental Practice Path

Congratulations, you've conquered dental school! But the journey doesn't end there. Now, a new adventure awaits: transitioning from student to independent practitioner. While exciting, this leap can be filled with uncertainties. Fear not, this book is your compass, guiding you through the intricate process of opening and managing your own dental practice.

Bridging the Gap

Remember those late-night anatomy sessions? Dental school honed your clinical skills, but may not have prepared you for the entrepreneurial side of dentistry. This book bridges that gap, providing practical insights and actionable advice to navigate the complexities of running your own business.

Embrace Your Independence

Forget punching a clock! Being your own boss means charting your own course. This book empowers you to make informed decisions about patient care, practice direction, and your overall career. Remember, autonomy equals long-term satisfaction and success.

Navigating the Modern Maze

From cutting-edge technology to digital marketing, the dental landscape is ever-evolving. Here, you'll find the knowledge and tools to stay ahead of the curve. Learn how to incorporate AI, adapt your marketing strategies, and position your practice for success in the modern medical ecosystem.

The Entrepreneurial Spirit:

Opening a practice requires more than just technical know-how; it demands resourcefulness and creativity. This book cultivates that entrepreneurial mindset, instilling business acumen, financial literacy, and strategic thinking. With these tools, you'll approach challenges with resilience and a proactive spirit.

Preserving the Core

Amidst the business hustle, never forget the essence of dentistry – *the patient.* This book emphasizes prioritizing patient-centric care, fostering a warm and welcoming atmosphere, and upholding ethical standards. Remember, entrepreneurship should enhance, not compromise, your core values.

Crafting Your Journey

No two dentists are alike, and neither are their aspirations. Whether you dream of a solo practice, a partnership, or exploring alternative models, this book provides adaptable guidance. Tailor the insights to your individual goals and circumstances, creating a personalized roadmap to success.

From Grad to Go

This book is your companion on the journey from graduation to practice ownership. With practical advice, real-world examples, and a focus on the entrepreneurial spirit, it empowers you to shape your path, preserving the essence of dentistry while thriving in the modern healthcare landscape. Remember, this is your journey, own it!

3. The Choice Between Startup vs an Acquisition

Choosing between starting your own dental practice and purchasing an existing one is a deeply personal odyssey—one that resonates with the heartbeat of your professional aspirations. As healthcare providers, the allure of an established practice often casts a tempting shadow, seemingly shielding us from the uncertainties inherent in starting afresh. However, what if I were to propose that forging your own path could unveil a more fulfilling and less perilous journey?

In the domain of purchasing an existing practice, the evaluation typically centers on tangible metrics like revenue and earnings, often neglecting nuanced factors such as the age of equipment and the intricate dynamics among staff members. However, as we stand on the brink of a digital revolution in healthcare, there's a pressing need to embrace transformative technologies—a departure from conventional practices of the past.

Consider, too, the stealthy attrition that often follows a purchase—a gradual exodus of patients that isn't merely a numerical decline but inflicts a substantial financial toll. However, the true epiphany awaits within the domain of startups. Yes, there are initial hurdles to surmount, including cash flow challenges. However, therein lies the allure—the freedom to harness modern tools and fashion, a practice that bears the imprint of your unique identity. Embarking on the journey of starting your own practice is akin to sculpting a legacy—a sanctuary that reflects your vision, rather than a mere continuation of someone else's narrative. While corporate dentistry may view each office as a mere cog in the profit wheel, your own practice transcends mere financial metrics. It becomes an extension of your essence—a sanctuary where the personal touch reigns supreme, and your commitment to your patients transcends the confines of a job description.

Indeed, the initial stages of a startup may be fraught with challenges, including the ever-looming specter of cash flow woes. Yet, the sheer satisfaction of witnessing your vision unfurl and flourish is unparalleled. It's the human factor—the palpable connection forged with your patients—that imbues your journey with purpose and meaning. In embracing the embryonic stages of your practice, you lay the foundation for exponential growth and fulfillment over the long haul.

Your dental office isn't merely a place of work—it's your sanctuary, your testament to passion, and the beating heart of your professional legacy. Embrace the uncertainties, relish the journey, and behold as your vision transforms into an enduring testament to your courage and conviction.

II

Self-Assessment and Goal Setting

1. Identifying Personal and Professional Goals

Launching your own dental practice is an exciting, yet daunting, adventure. Beyond clinical expertise, crafting a fulfilling and successful career requires setting meaningful goals that reflect both your personal aspirations and professional ambitions. This chapter acts as your guide, exploring the intricate connections between these two domains and offering practical strategies to translate your vision into reality.

The Intertwined Threads

Imagine yourself standing at a crossroads, where personal and professional paths converge. Here, your values, beliefs, and passions intertwine with your career aspirations, shaping the future of your practice. Consider how your dedication to empathy, integrity, and community involvement can blossom into the unique ethos of your clinic, fostering trust and connection with patients and staff alike.

Unearthing Your Personal Compass

Before embarking on the goal-setting adventure, embark on a journey of *self-discovery*. Ask yourself: what core values guide me? How do they influence my approach to patient care and interpersonal relationships? By unraveling your personal values, you lay the foundation for a practice that authentically reflects your beliefs, fostering trust and connection with your team and patients.

From Dream to SMART Reality

Transform vague aspirations into tangible objectives using the SMART framework. **Specific**, **Measurable**, **Achievable**, **Relevant**, and **Time-bound** goals offer a clear roadmap for your career journey. Craft short-term goals, like building a solid patient base or streamlining administrative processes, alongside long-term ambitions like practice expansion and multi-location.

Finding Harmony

Remember, professional success should never come at the expense of personal well-being. Strike a balance between your ambitions in both realms, ensuring that your pursuit of dental excellence integrates seamlessly with a fulfilling personal life. Identify potential challenges and embrace strategies for maintaining equilibrium, fostering sustainable success and satisfaction.

Living Your Goals, Each Day

Goal-setting isn't just about theoretical aspirations; it's about weaving your objectives into the daily fabric of your practice. Explore how patient interactions, team meetings, and business decisions align with your overarching goals. This alignment not only provides direction but infuses your daily work with purpose, creating a meaningful and cohesive practice environment.

Embrace the Dynamic Journey

Remember, your goals are living entities, evolving alongside your circumstances. Regularly assess your progress, celebrate milestones, and be open to adapting them as needed. This agility embodies resilience, a crucial trait in the ever-changing landscape of dental practice ownership.

Your Practice, Your Purpose:

The entrepreneurial journey in dentistry begins with a clear understanding and alignment of personal and professional goals. This chapter serves as your compass, guiding you towards a practice that not only thrives financially but also resonates with your deeper sense of purpose and fulfillment. As you embark on this transformative journey, remember that your goals are the foundation upon which you build a flourishing and authentic practice, reflecting your unique vision and values.

2. Assessing Financial Readiness

Launching a dental practice is thrilling, but navigating the financial aspects can feel like scaling Mount Everest in flip-flops. Fear not, intrepid dentist! This chapter equips you with the knowledge and tools to build a robust financial fortress, ensuring your practice strives for years to come.

Mapping Your Territory: Understanding the Financial Landscape

Imagine your dental startup as a castle. To defend it, you need to know the surrounding terrain. This means meticulously mapping your financial landscape – startup costs (building lease, equipment, technology), ongoing expenses (payroll, supplies, marketing), and potential revenue streams (patient fees, insurance contracts). Don't rely on guesswork; research, forecast, and create a detailed financial plan. This map becomes your blueprint for informed decisions, ensuring your fortress remains financially secure.

Taming the Student Loan Dragon: Strategies for Debt Management

Student loan debt looms large for many graduates, like a fire-breathing dragon guarding your path. Assess your loans – understand their terms, interest rates, and repayment options. Explore strategies like income-driven repayment plans or consolidation to ensure these loans don't become an insurmountable obstacle. Consider seeking professional financial advice; a wise advisor can be your knight in shining armor, helping you slay the debt dragon and clear the path to financial freedom.

Building Your Budgetary Bulwark: Creating a Sustainable Cash Flow

Your personal budget is the foundation of your financial fortress. Learn how to build one that aligns your income with expenses like rent, groceries, and yes, those pesky loan payments. Use budgeting apps and practical tips to become a master of resource allocation, ensuring your personal finances are healthy. Remember, a strong personal budget directly supports the financial well-being of your practice.

Choosing Your Financial Arsenal: Exploring Funding Options

Funding your practice requires selecting the right weapons from your arsenal. Options include traditional loans, angel investors, and even government grants. Each comes with its advantages and risks. Analyze your risk tolerance and financial goals to choose the best fit for your battle plan. We will discuss financing options in the next chapters.

Remember: Financial preparedness is an ongoing quest, not a one-time victory. By meticulously mapping your territory, taming the student loan dragon, building your budgetary bulwark, choosing the right financial weapons, and learning from the battle-tested, you set your practice up for long-term success. This chapter empowers you with the financial literacy needed to make informed decisions and ensure your practice not only survives but flourishes in the dynamic realm of dental entrepreneurship. So grab your financial sword and shield, charge into the future with confidence, and build a practice that will stand strong for years to come!

3. Setting Goals and Building your Team

Launching your own dental practice isn't just about financial success; it's about building something meaningful and aligned with your deepest aspirations. This chapter is your guide to goal alignment, a powerful tool that transforms your dreams into a thriving and impactful practice.

Craft Your Practice's Story:

Imagine your practice as a unique story waiting to be told. What are the core values and principles that will define its chapters? Do you envision a warm, welcoming environment focused on building patient relationships? Or a tech-driven practice offering cutting-edge treatments? Articulating your vision provides a roadmap for setting goals that bring your unique story to life.

Values: The Heart of Your Practice Culture:

Think of your core values as the beating heart of your practice. How will your commitment to compassion, integrity, or community involvement weave into the fabric of your daily operations? Infuse these values into your team culture, patient interactions, and even marketing materials. When your practice reflects your values, it fosters authenticity and attracts patients who share your vision.

From Dream to Action: Strategic Planning for Success:

Strategic planning bridges the gap between your vision and reality. Imagine breaking down your overall vision into achievable milestones like increasing the patient base by 10% within a year or implementing a new patient education program. Set SMART goals that are specific, measurable, achievable, relevant, and time-bound. This strategic plan becomes your actionable roadmap, guiding you towards your ultimate destination.

Embrace the Evolving Landscape:

Dentistry is dynamic! New technologies, changing patient expectations, and evolving industry trends can impact your practice in unexpected ways. Staying adaptable ensures your goals remain relevant. Research emerging trends like tele-dentistry or personalized medicine, and consider how they might fit into your vision. By embracing change, you ensure your practice continues to thrive in an ever-shifting landscape. Aligning your personal and professional goals with your practice's vision is a journey, not a destination. By crafting a compelling narrative, infusing your values, strategically planning, and embracing adaptability, you build a fulfilling and impactful practice. Remember, this chapter is your guide, empowering you to navigate the exciting journey of shaping your dental practice dream into a vibrant reality. So, grab your compass, set your course, and watch your vision unfold!

Building your Team:

Embarking on a dental practice startup journey can feel like a daunting task, but you are not alone in this endeavor. In fact, you have the opportunity to assemble a team of dedicated professionals who specialize in guiding entrepreneurs like yourself through every step of the process. These individuals are seasoned experts who understand the ins and outs of the dental industry and are committed to helping you achieve your goals. Whether you find them online, through consultancy firms, or through referrals, rest assured that they are there to provide invaluable support and expertise.

Working with a team of professionals not only streamlines the startup process but also fosters a sense of collaboration and camaraderie. You'll find that these individuals are not just service providers; they are trusted partners who are genuinely invested in your success. They will go above and beyond to address your concerns, answer your questions, and offer creative solutions to any obstacles you may encounter along the way.

As you engage with your dream team, you'll have the opportunity to meet a diverse array of individuals, each with their own unique talents and perspectives. From the meticulous attention to detail of your attorney to the innovative design concepts of your architect, you'll be inspired by the passion and dedication of those you collaborate with. Together, you'll celebrate victories, overcome challenges, and ultimately, bring your vision of a thriving dental practice to life. Here is a list of your team of professionals:

- **Bank Representative**: Assists with the loan application process, financial analysis, and funding arrangements for the dental practice startup.
- **Bank Underwriter**: Evaluates the financial viability and creditworthiness of the dental practice loan application, assessing risk factors and determining loan terms and conditions.
- **Real Estate Broker**: Helps identify and secure a suitable property for the dental office, considering factors such as location, size, zoning regulations, and lease or purchase terms.
- **Attorney**: Provides legal guidance on lease negotiations, entity formation (e.g., LLC setup), contracts, compliance issues, and other legal matters related to the establishment of the dental practice.
- **Architect or Designer**: Collaborates with you to plan and design the layout of the office space, ensuring optimal functionality, compliance with regulations, and an inviting patient environment.
- **General Contractor**: Oversees the construction or renovation of the dental office space, managing subcontractors, timelines, and budget to ensure the project's successful completion.
- **Equipment Specialist**: Assists in selecting and procuring dental equipment, technology, and furnishings for the practice, ensuring they meet the specific needs and budget of the practice.

- **Insurance Agent/Broker**: Helps obtain necessary insurance coverage for the dental practice, including liability, malpractice, property, and business interruption insurance.
- **IT Specialist**: Sets up and maintains the practice's technology infrastructure, including computer systems, software, cybersecurity measures, and electronic health records (EHR) systems.
- **Marketing Consultant/Agency:** Develops and implements marketing strategies to promote the dental practice, attract new patients, and build brand awareness in the local community.
- **Practice Management Consultant**: Provides guidance on staff training, workflow optimization, patient experience enhancement, and overall practice management strategies to maximize efficiency and profitability.
- **Human Resources Consultant**: Assists with staffing, employee relations, compliance with labor laws, HR policies, and procedures to create a positive and productive work environment.
- **Dental Laboratory Technician:** Collaborates with the dental practice to fabricate custom dental prosthetics, restorations, and appliances, ensuring quality and timely delivery of dental lab services.
- **Accountant/Financial Advisor:** Offers financial planning, budgeting, tax planning, and business structuring advice to ensure financial stability and compliance with regulatory requirements.

By assembling a comprehensive team of professionals, the dental practice owner can navigate the complexities of starting a new practice with confidence and expertise, setting the stage for long-term success and growth.

III

Legal and Regulatory Steps

1. Licensing and Credentialing

Opening your dream dental practice requires more than just a drill and a dazzling smile. Before welcoming patients, you need to conquer the complex yet crucial world of licensing and credentialing. This chapter acts as your map, guiding you through the labyrinth of requirements and procedures to establish your practice on solid legal and professional ground.

Understanding Licensing Requirements

Every state has its own unique set of rules for dentists. This section demystifies the common elements of licensing, including:

- **Dental License:** To practice dentistry, you need to obtain a dental license from the state's dental board. This typically involves completing an accredited dental program, passing written and practical exams, and fulfilling any other requirements set by the state board.

- **Business License:** You will likely need a general business license to operate any business, including a dental practice. This can usually be obtained from your city or county government.
- **Professional Corporation**: Many states require healthcare professionals, including dentists, to form a professional corporation or limited liability company (LLC) to operate their practice. This provides certain legal protections and tax benefits.
- **DEA Registration**: If you will be prescribing controlled substances, you'll need to register with the Drug Enforcement Administration (DEA).
- **Malpractice Insurance**: Most states require dentists to carry malpractice insurance to protect themselves and their patients in case of any legal claims.
- **Health Department Permits**: Depending on the services you offer, you may need permits or inspections from the local health department to ensure compliance with health and safety regulations.
- **HIPAA Compliance**: Dental practices must comply with the Health Insurance Portability and Accountability Act (HIPAA) regulations regarding patient privacy and data security.
- **Zoning and Building Permits**: You'll need to ensure that your office location complies with local zoning laws and obtain any necessary building permits for renovations or construction.
- **Employer Identification Number (EIN)**: You'll need to obtain an EIN from the IRS for tax purposes, especially if you plan to hire employees.

- **Business Insurance**: In addition to malpractice insurance, you may need other types of business insurance, such as property insurance and liability insurance, to protect your practice from unexpected events.
- **Continuing Education**: Many states require dentists to complete a certain number of hours of continuing education each year to maintain their license.
- **Infection Control Compliance**: You'll need to follow infection control protocols set by the Centers for Disease Control and Prevention (CDC) and other regulatory agencies to prevent the spread of infections in your practice.

Claiming Your Unique Number: Acquiring Your National Provider Identifier (NPI)

In starting a dental office, getting a National Provider Identifier (NPI) is crucial. This unique ID is needed for billing, identifying patients, and making administrative tasks easier. To obtain an NPI for your dental office:

- Visit the NPI Enumerator Website: Access the National Plan and Provider Enumeration System (NPPES) website, which serves as the platform for applying for an NPI. You can find it at https://nppes.cms.hhs.gov.
- Create an Account: Register for an account on the NPPES website if you haven't already. You'll need to provide some basic information and create login credentials.
- Complete the Application: Log in to your account and fill out the NPI application form. This form will ask for details about your dental office, including its name, address, contact information, and tax identification number (TIN).

- Select the Type of NPI: Choose the appropriate type of NPI for your dental office. For a dental practice, this will likely be a Type 2 NPI, which is assigned to healthcare providers and organizations.
- Provide Additional Information: You may need to provide additional information about your practice, such as the types of services you offer and any affiliations with other healthcare providers or organizations.
- Review and Submit: Review the information you've provided for accuracy and completeness. Once you're satisfied, submit the application.
- Wait for Processing: After submitting the application, you'll need to wait for it to be processed. This typically takes a few business days, but it can vary depending on the volume of applications being processed.
- Receive Your NPI: Once your application has been processed and approved, you'll receive your NPI via email or mail. Make sure to keep this number in a secure place, as you'll need it for various administrative tasks related to your dental practice.

Becoming a Player in the Insurance Landscape: Credentialing with Providers

Expanding your patient base often hinges on accepting insurance. These are the general credentialing steps:

- **Gather Required Information**: Collect all necessary documentation and information required for credentialing. This typically includes your dental license, DEA registration, malpractice insurance information, office location details, tax identification number, and any other relevant business documents.

- **Select Insurance Plans**: Decide which insurance plans the dental office wishes to accept. This decision may depend on factors such as patient demographics, geographic location, and the preferences of the dental practice.
- **Complete Applications**: Obtain credentialing applications for the selected insurance plans. These applications can usually be obtained directly from the insurance companies or through their websites. Complete all sections of the applications accurately and thoroughly. Submit the completed applications to the insurance companies either electronically or via mail, following their specific submission instructions. Ensure that all required documents and information are included with each application to avoid delays in the credentialing process.
- **Follow-Up**: After submitting the applications, follow up with the insurance companies to confirm receipt and to inquire about the status of the credentialing process. Be prepared to provide any additional information or documentation requested by the insurance companies.
- **Provider Enrollment**: Once the insurance companies have reviewed the applications and approved the dental office for participation in their networks, the next step is provider enrollment. This involves completing additional enrollment forms and agreements to officially become a participating provider with each insurance plan.
- **Contract Review**: Carefully review the terms and conditions of the provider contracts offered by the insurance plans. Pay close attention to reimbursement rates, payment schedules, coverage limitations, and any other contractual obligations.
- **Negotiation**: If there are aspects of the provider contracts that you wish to negotiate, such as reimbursement rates or

contractual terms, engage in negotiations with the insurance companies to reach mutually acceptable agreements.

- **Execute Contracts**: Once any negotiations are complete and both parties agree to the terms, sign the provider contracts and return them to the insurance companies as instructed.
- **Receive Confirmation**: Upon receipt of the signed contracts, the insurance companies will typically provide written confirmation of the dental office's participation in their networks. This confirmation may include details such as effective dates of participation and any additional requirements or steps to be completed.
- **Update Systems and Staff**: Ensure that all office systems, billing software, and staff members are updated with the necessary information to begin accepting patients covered by the newly credentialed insurance plans.
- **Monitor and Maintain Credentials**: Regularly monitor the status of provider credentials with each insurance plan to ensure ongoing compliance with their requirements. This may involve renewing credentials periodically and updating information as needed.

In-Network vs Out of Network Status:

In-network participation offers new dental practices increased patient accessibility and simplified reimbursements. By joining relevant insurance networks, practices attract more patients seeking reduced out-of-pocket costs and benefit from pre-negotiated fees, streamlining revenue management and administrative tasks.

Advantages of In-Network Status :

- **Maximized Patient Accessibility**: Being in-network expands the patient base as individuals covered by the insurance plans associated with the practice can access services with reduced out-of-pocket costs.
- **Streamlined Reimbursements**: In-network participation entails pre-negotiated fees for services, ensuring predictable revenue streams and simplified billing processes.
- **Enhanced Practice Visibility**: Listing as an in-network provider can attract more patients, bolstering the practice's reputation and facilitating a steady influx of clientele.
- **Access to Support Services**: Insurance companies typically offer online portals and dedicated representatives to assist with claims processing and administrative tasks, reducing the practice's workload.

Disadvantages of In-Network Status:

- **Limited Fee Control**: In-network providers must adhere to the reimbursement rates set by insurance companies, potentially resulting in lower fees for services compared to out-of-network providers.
- **Contractual Obligations**: Providers may be subject to contractual terms and conditions imposed by insurance companies, including network restrictions and coverage limitations.
- **Potential for Lower Reimbursement**: While in-network participation offers predictability, reimbursement rates may still be lower compared to what could be charged as an out-of-network provider.

- **Dependency on Insurance Companies**: Practices may become reliant on insurance networks, limiting flexibility in setting fees and managing patient populations.

Advantages of Out-of-Network Status:

- **Greater Fee Flexibility**: Out-of-network providers have more control over setting their fees, potentially allowing for higher reimbursement rates for services rendered.
- **Autonomy in Decision-Making**: Practices can operate independently without being bound by the terms and conditions imposed by insurance networks, retaining greater control over patient care and business operations.
- **Potential for Higher Reimbursement**: Without contractual constraints, out-of-network providers may receive higher reimbursement rates for services provided to patients.
- **Reduced Dependency on Insurance Companies**: Practices can diversify their revenue streams by attracting patients who are willing to pay out-of-network rates, reducing reliance on insurance networks.

Disadvantages of Out-of-Network Status:

- **Limited Patient Pool**: Being out-of-network may deter patients seeking reduced out-of-pocket costs, potentially limiting the practice's clientele and market reach.
- **Increased Patient Responsibility**: Patients may incur higher out-of-pocket expenses when receiving services from

out-of-network providers, leading to potential dissatisfaction or financial strain.

Outsourcing credentialing tasks to a specialized service company offers dental offices a streamlined process by leveraging the company's expertise, efficiency, and dedicated resources. These companies navigate complex insurance network requirements, expedite credentialing turnaround times, and ensure compliance with regulations, freeing up dental office staff to focus on essential practice management tasks. By managing documentation, facilitating communication with insurance companies, and providing regular updates, credentialing service companies mitigate administrative burdens and minimize delays, ultimately leading to a quicker start in accepting patients and generating revenue. Though there's a cost involved, the benefits in terms of time saved, accuracy, and compliance often justify the investment, making it a cost-effective solution for dental practices aiming to efficiently navigate the credentialing process.

2. Choosing a Legal Structure

Forming an LLC and Obtaining an EIN

Launching your dental practice isn't just about clinical skills; it's about building a sustainable business from the ground up. Selecting the right legal structure is a crucial first step, impacting liability, taxation, and your overall flexibility. This chapter guides you through the process of forming a Limited Liability Company (LLC), a popular choice for dental practices, and obtaining your crucial Employer Identification Number (EIN).

Why Choose an LLC?

Imagine your dental practice as a castle. An LLC acts as a sturdy wall, shielding your personal assets from business liabilities. Unlike being a sole proprietor, if someone sues your practice, they can only go after the business's assets, not your personal savings or home. Beyond protection, LLCs offer:

- **Pass-through Taxation**: This means your business profits and losses "pass through" to your personal tax return, avoiding double taxation.
- **Management Flexibility**: Choose how you want to manage your practice – as a single owner, with partners, or even employees. An operating agreement outlines these details.
- **Simplified Administration**: Compared to corporations, LLCs require less paperwork and fewer formalities.

Building Your LLC Castle: Step-by-Step Guide

- **Pick Your Banner**: Choose a unique business name that complies with state regulations. Check availability and register it officially.
- **Lay the Foundation**: File Articles of Organization with your state's appropriate agency. This document contains basic information about your LLC.
- **Appoint Your Guardian**: Designate a Registered Agent to receive legal documents on your LLC's behalf. This could be a person or a service.

- **Define Your Laws**: Create an Operating Agreement. This sets the rules for running your LLC, including ownership percentages, profits/losses distribution, and voting rights. While not always mandatory, it's highly recommended for clarity and future ease.
- **Obtain Permits and Licenses**: Check what additional licenses or permits are required for dental practices in your state and ensure you have them.

Acquiring Your EIN: The Business Key

Think of your EIN as a unique key that unlocks various business opportunities. You'll need it for:

- **Opening a business bank account**: Separate your personal and business finances for clarity and legal protection.
- **Hiring employees**: Report payroll taxes and file relevant forms.
- **Filing business taxes**: Pay federal and state taxes according to your LLC structure.

Getting Your EIN is Easy:

- Visit the IRS website and access the online EIN application portal.
- Carefully complete the application, providing details about your LLC, ownership, and how you'll use the EIN.
- Upon successful application, you'll receive your EIN immediately.

Forming your LLC and obtaining your EIN are crucial first steps. Remember to:

- **Open a Business Bank Account**: Use your EIN to establish a separate bank account for your practice's financial transactions.
- **Seek Tax Guidance**: Consult a tax professional to understand your LLC's tax implications and plan accordingly.
- **Maintain Compliance**: Stay updated on state and federal regulations and file necessary reports to keep your LLC in good standing.

Choosing an LLC and obtaining an EIN are essential steps in building a strong foundation for your dental practice. By following these guidelines and seeking professional advice when needed, you'll set your business up for success, navigate legal requirements smoothly, and focus on what matters most - delivering exceptional dental care to your patients!

3. Navigating Healthcare Regulations and Compliance

While grand visions and clinical expertise are crucial, a strong foundation built on compliance with healthcare regulations is paramount. This chapter equips you, the intrepid dental practitioner, with the knowledge and tools to navigate the complex, yet essential, world of regulations.

Safeguarding Patient Privacy: The Fortress of HIPAA

Think of HIPAA (Health Insurance Portability and Accountability Act) as the impenetrable walls protecting your patients' confidential information. Delve into:

- The Core: Understand the fundamental principles of HIPAA, emphasizing patient privacy and security within your practice.
- Building Your Defenses: Implement robust HIPAA policies and procedures, covering topics like data access, patient communication, and breach response plans. Train your team to be vigilant guardians of patient privacy.
- Securing the Digital Realm: Explore data security measures like encryption, secure email practices, and regular backups to safeguard electronic health records (EHRs) and other sensitive information. Remember, data breaches can be costly and damaging.

A Sanctuary of Safety: Upholding OSHA Standards

Imagine OSHA (Occupational Safety and Health Administration) as the guardians, ensuring a safe and healthy work environment for you and your team. Explore:

- OSHA in Dentistry: Understand the specific regulations governing dental practices, prioritizing employee safety and well-being.
- Infection Control: Your Armor: Master sterilization protocols, proper use of personal protective equipment (PPE), and waste disposal procedures to minimize exposure risks.
- Beyond Infection Control: Address broader safety aspects like ergonomics, fire safety, and hazardous materials handling,

creating a culture of safety that permeates your entire practice.

Self-Assessment: The Vigilant Knight

Just like knights regularly inspected their armor, periodic internal audits assess your compliance with regulations. Embrace self-assessment to:

- **Identify vulnerabilities**: Regularly evaluate your practice's adherence to HIPAA, OSHA, and billing guidelines.
- **Mitigate risks**: Address any shortcomings promptly, preventing potential penalties and ensuring continuous improvement.
- **Stay proactive**: Remain vigilant by conducting regular training for your team and seeking professional guidance when needed.

The Ever-Shifting Landscape: Adapting to Change

Regulations are like a flowing river, constantly evolving. To stay ahead of the curve:

- **Become a Knowledge Seeker**: Subscribe to reliable healthcare compliance resources to stay informed about regulatory updates and changes.
- **Proactive Integration**: Adapt your practice policies and procedures promptly to align with evolving regulations, demonstrating your commitment to compliance.

Navigating healthcare regulations and compliance may seem daunting, but like building a flourishing practice, it's an essential journey. By understanding key regulations like HIPAA, OSHA, and insurance guidelines, and adopting practices like self-assessment and continuous learning, you build a practice on solid ground. Remember, prioritizing patient safety, data security, and legal integrity is not just about compliance, it's about building trust and fostering a thriving dental practice. This chapter empowers you to embark on this journey with confidence, knowing you have the knowledge and tools to navigate the regulatory landscape and emerge as a true champion of ethical and compliant dental care.

IV

Financial Planning

1. Estimating Startup Costs

Launching a successful dental practice requires more than just clinical expertise; it demands strategic financial planning to ensure sustainability and growth. This chapter provides essential insights to help you navigate the financial aspects of starting your practice, from estimating startup costs to managing ongoing expenses effectively.

Every dental practice startup is unique, with startup costs varying based on the type and scale of the practice you envision. Consider the following key factors when estimating startup costs:

Location Strategy: Lease vs. Own

Choosing the right physical space is a pivotal decision. Evaluate the benefits of leasing for flexibility and cost-effectiveness versus the long-term stability and potential investment returns of ownership. Analyze local market dynamics, growth projections, and financial resources to make an informed choice aligned with your practice vision.

Advantages of Leasing a Dental Office:

- **Lower Initial Costs**: Leasing typically requires less upfront capital compared to purchasing a property, making it more accessible for new dental practitioners with limited funds.
- **Flexibility**: Leasing offers flexibility in terms of location and space size, allowing dentists to easily relocate or expand their practice as needed without the financial commitment of owning.
- **Reduced Maintenance Responsibilities**: The landlord is generally responsible for property maintenance and repairs, relieving the tenant of the burden and costs associated with property upkeep.

Disadvantages of Leasing a Dental Office:

- **Lack of Equity**: Unlike owning a property, leasing does not build equity, meaning dentists miss out on potential long-term investment gains and asset appreciation.
- Rent Increases: Lease agreements may include rent escalation clauses, allowing landlords to raise rent periodically, potentially leading to higher operating costs over time.
- **Limited Control**: Tenants have limited control over the property, with restrictions on renovations, alterations, and customization to suit the practice's specific needs and preferences.
- **Uncertainty**: Leasing is subject to the terms and conditions of the lease agreement, which may change at the landlord's

discretion, leading to uncertainty and potential instability for the dental practice.

Advantages of Owning the Property:

- **Equity Building**: Ownership allows dentists to build equity in the property over time, providing potential long-term financial benefits and asset appreciation.
- Control and Customization: Property ownership grants full control over the space, enabling dentists to customize and design the office layout to meet their unique preferences and practice requirements.
- **Stability and Predictability**: Owning a property offers stability and predictability in terms of occupancy costs, as mortgage payments remain consistent over the loan term, providing greater financial security for the dental practice.
- **Investment Potential:** Property ownership presents opportunities for additional income streams, such as leasing out unused space to other tenants or selling the property for a profit in the future.

Disadvantages of Owning the Property:

- **Higher Initial Costs:** Purchasing a property typically requires a significant upfront investment, including down payments, closing costs, and ongoing mortgage payments, which may be challenging for new practitioners or those with limited funds.
- **Maintenance Responsibilities**: Property owners are responsible for property maintenance, repairs, and upkeep,

which can be costly and time-consuming, especially for older buildings or unforeseen issues.

- **Limited Flexibility**: Ownership ties dentists to a specific location and property, reducing flexibility to relocate or expand the practice without selling or leasing the property.
- **Market Risks**: Property values and market conditions are subject to fluctuations, posing potential risks and uncertainties for property owners in terms of investment returns and property appreciation.

2. Budgeting for Construction and Renovation

Embarking on the construction or renovation of your dental practice space requires meticulous planning and budgeting to ensure a smooth and cost-effective process. Whether you're starting from scratch or revamping an existing space, here are essential steps to consider:

Architectural and Design Fees:

- Initial consultation and concept development
- Detailed architectural drawings and plans
- Interior design and layout services

Permitting and Regulatory Costs:

- Building permits
- Zoning variances, if applicable
- Compliance with local building codes and regulations

Construction Materials:

- Structural materials (e.g., steel, concrete)
- Framing and drywall
- Flooring materials (e.g., tiles, laminate)
- Ceiling materials (e.g., acoustic tiles)
- Insulation and soundproofing materials

Contractor Fees and Labor Costs:

- General contractor fees
- Construction labor costs (carpenters, electricians, plumbers, etc.)
- Project management fees

Mechanical and Electrical Systems:

- HVAC (heating, ventilation, air conditioning) systems
- Plumbing and drainage systems
- Electrical wiring and lighting fixtures

Dental Equipment and Technology:

- Dental chairs and operatories
- X-ray machines and imaging equipment
- Sterilization equipment
- Computers, servers, and networking infrastructure
- Software systems (practice management software, electronic health records)

Furnishings and Fixtures:

- Reception area furniture
- Waiting room seating
- Cabinetry and storage solutions
- Office desks and chairs
- Decorative fixtures and accessories

Safety and Security Systems:

- Fire alarm and sprinkler systems
- Security cameras and surveillance equipment
- Access control systems (key cards, biometric scanners)

Finishes and Décor:

- Paint and wall coverings
- Decorative finishes (e.g., wainscoting, crown molding)
- Window treatments
- Signage and branding

Contingency Fund:

Reserve for unexpected expenses and contingencies (e.g., unforeseen construction delays, change orders, cost overruns)

It's essential to work closely with your architect, contractor, and other professionals to develop a comprehensive budget that accounts for all aspects of your dental practice construction project. Be sure to regularly monitor expenses and adjust your budget as needed to ensure that your project stays on track and within budget.

Optimal Number of Operatories:

When considering the number of operatories for your dental practice, it's wise to start small and scale up as needed. While leasing a space with 7-8 operatories may seem tempting, it's not necessary to have them all operational from day one. In the initial years, focusing on 3-4 operatories can effectively meet patient demand and ensure optimal workflow efficiency. This approach allows you to manage costs and resources more effectively, especially if you're not catering to a Medicaid-based clientele. However, it's essential to choose a space that can accommodate future growth, particularly if you plan to bring in an associate or expand your services down the line. By starting small and planning for scalability, you can adapt to evolving patient needs and ensure long-term success for your dental practice.

Marketing Investment: Building Your Brand

Recognizing the pivotal role of marketing in your practice's success, allocating resources towards strategic marketing initiatives is paramount. Allocate funds towards comprehensive endeavors such as website development, targeted advertising campaigns, and brand-building initiatives to solidify your practice's presence within the community. It's imperative to acknowledge that effective marketing is not a one-time endeavor but rather an ongoing commitment. Embrace sustainable strategies that ensure consistency and longevity in your marketing efforts, ultimately cultivating lasting relationships with patients and establishing your practice as a trusted healthcare provider within the community.

Working Capital Management: Ensuring Financial Stability

Launching a new dental practice comes with inherent uncertainties. It's essential to proactively allocate a portion of your budget towards working capital to effectively manage operational expenses such as payroll, utilities, and supplies during the initial phase. By establishing a robust financial safety net, you can navigate unforeseen challenges with confidence, ensuring uninterrupted operations and safeguarding against potential disruptions.

Summary of cost checklist

1. Lease or Mortgage Payments:

- Monthly lease payments or mortgage installments for your practice space.
- Construction or Renovation Costs: Permitting fees, architectural design, and contractor fees. Building materials, labor costs, and construction equipment rentals.
- Renovation of existing space or construction of a new facility.

2. Equipment and Technology Purchases:

- Dental chairs, X-ray machines, sterilization equipment, and dental instruments.
- Computer hardware, software systems (e.g., practice management software, electronic health records), and networking infrastructure.
- Dental technology and digital equipment for diagnostics and treatment planning.

3. Licenses and Permits:

- Fees for obtaining professional licenses, dental practice permits, and business registrations.
- Compliance fees for health and safety regulations, building codes, and zoning requirements.

4. **Initial Inventory:**

- Dental supplies (e.g., disposable gloves, masks, gauze, syringes, restorative materials).
- Office supplies (e.g., stationery, printer ink, cleaning supplies).
- Patient education materials, brochures, and promotional items.

5. **Marketing and Advertising Expenses:**

- Website development and maintenance.
- Digital marketing campaigns (e.g., social media advertising, Google Ads).
- Printed materials (e.g., brochures, business cards, flyers).
- Branding and logo design.

6. **Working Capital Reserve:**

- Funds set aside to cover operational expenses during the initial phase of the practice.
- Includes payroll, rent, utilities, insurance premiums, and other ongoing expenses.

7. **Professional Consultation Fees:**

- Fees for legal, accounting, and financial consulting services.

- Expert advice on business structure, tax planning, and financial management.

8. Contingency Fund for Unexpected Expenses:

- Reserve funds for unforeseen expenses, emergencies, and unexpected costs.
- Allows for flexibility in case of construction delays, equipment malfunctions, or other unexpected challenges.

Estimating startup costs isn't about guessing; it's about meticulous planning. By analyzing location options, managing construction costs, finding the right number of operatories, investing in marketing, building working capital, seeking expert guidance, and planning for contingencies, you create a comprehensive budget that sets your dental practice on a path to financial stability and success. Remember, this chapter is your guide, but your journey requires careful research, planning, and adaptation. With a realistic budget and a spirit of entrepreneurship, you can turn your dream practice into a thriving reality.

3. Creating a Comprehensive Budget for your Operation

Launching your dental practice requires not only top-notch clinical skills but also the wisdom of a financial architect. This chapter equips you with the tools and insights to craft a comprehensive budget, your foundation for long-term financial stability and growth.

Laying the Bricks: Categorizing Expenses

Imagine your budget as a sturdy wall, built with distinct bricks. First, categorize your expenses:

- **Fixed Costs**: Rent, utilities, loan payments – these remain constant month-to-month.
- **Variable Costs**: Supplies, marketing, staff overtime – these fluctuate based on activity.

The Operational Heartbeat: Managing Day-to-Day Variable Expenses

- **Optimizing Expenses**: Implement cost-saving strategies without compromising patient care. Negotiate bills, explore efficient suppliers, and utilize technology for streamlining processes.
- **Accurate Projections**: Forecast expenses based on historical data and market trends to ensure smooth day-to-day operations.

Sowing the Seeds for Growth: Marketing and Expansion

Investing in marketing is like planting seeds for patient growth. Allocate funds for:

- **Building a Brand**: Develop a strong brand identity through website design, logo creation, and consistent messaging.

- **Targeted Advertising**: Reach your ideal patients with strategic advertising campaigns across relevant channels.
- **Patient Engagement**: Implement initiatives to retain existing patients and build loyalty.

Staying Ahead of the Curve: Technology and Infrastructure

Technology isn't just a cost; it's an investment in the future. Allocate funds for:

- **Technology Maintenance**: Regular maintenance and upgrades ensure smooth operations and efficient patient care.
- **Embracing Innovation**: Consider investing in cutting-edge technologies to enhance patient experience and stay ahead of the competition.

Constant Vigilance: Regular Reviews and Adjustments

Think of budget reviews as regular check-ups on your financial health. Here's why they're crucial:

- Identify Variances: Compare actual expenses to projections and pinpoint areas needing adjustments.
- Make Informed Decisions: Use data-driven insights to optimize spending and allocate resources effectively.
- Adapt to Change: Remain flexible and adjust your budget as your practice evolves and market conditions shift.

Investing in the Future: Growth Strategies

Don't just plan for today; think about tomorrow. Allocate funds for:

- **Expanding Services**: Offer new services to attract a wider patient base.
- **Opening New Locations**: Strategically expand your reach by opening additional practice branches.
- **Innovative Technologies:** Invest in cutting-edge technologies to differentiate your practice and attract tech-savvy patients.

Financial Checkups: Periodic Assessments

Conducting regular financial assessments is like getting a comprehensive health screening for your practice. Explore:

- **Key Performance Indicators (KPIs)**: Track metrics like patient acquisition costs, average patient value, and treatment conversion rates to gauge performance.
- **Marketing ROI**: Evaluate the return on investment for your marketing initiatives to optimize campaign effectiveness.
- **Alignment with Goals**: Ensure your financial decisions align with your overall practice goals and long-term vision.

Demystifying financial statements:

In this chapter, we delve into the foundational trio of financial statements essential for businesses: the income statement, balance sheet, and cash flow statement. We explore their relevance and practical applications within the context of dentistry, elucidating how these financial tools can offer invaluable insights into the financial health and operational dynamics of dental practices.

- **The Income Statement:**

Purpose: The income statement, also known as the profit and loss statement, provides a snapshot of the dental office's financial performance over a specific period, typically monthly, quarterly, or annually. It details the revenues generated by the practice, the expenses incurred in generating those revenues, and the resulting net income or loss.

Importance: The income statement helps dental office managers assess the profitability of the practice, identify trends in revenue and expenses, and evaluate the effectiveness of financial management strategies. It provides valuable insights into the practice's revenue streams, cost structure, and overall financial health.

Revenue:	Patient Services Revenue: - Routine Check-ups - Cleanings - Dental Procedures - Other Patient Services Other Revenue: - Product Sales - Rental Income (if applicable) - Other Sources of Revenue **Total Revenue**
Cost of Goods Sold (COGS):	- Dental Supplies - Lab Fees - Other Direct Costs **Total Cost of Goods Sold**
Gross Profit:	= Revenue - Cost of Goods Sold
Operating Expenses:	- Rent - Utilities - Salaries and Benefits - Office Supplies - Marketing and Advertising - Equipment Maintenance - Professional Fees - Other Operating Expenses **Total Operating Expenses**
Net Operating Income (NOI):	= Gross Profit - Operating Expenses
Other Income and Expenses:	- Interest Income - Investment Gains/Losses - Taxes - Depreciation - Amortization - Other Income/Expenses **Total Other Income and Expenses**

The Income Statement

- **The Cash Flow Statement:**

Purpose: The cash flow statement tracks the inflows and outflows of cash in the dental office over a specific period. It categorizes cash transactions into three main categories: operating activities (e.g., revenue from patient services, payments for supplies), investing activities (e.g., purchases of equipment, investments), and financing activities (e.g., loans, equity financing).

Importance: The cash flow statement helps dental office managers monitor the liquidity and solvency of the practice by assessing its ability to generate and manage cash. It provides insights into the sources and uses of cash, helps identify cash flow trends and patterns, and enables proactive cash management to ensure the practice has sufficient liquidity to meet its financial obligations.

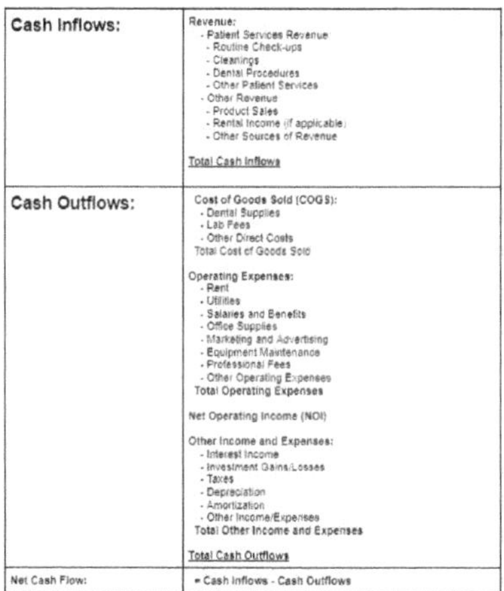

Cash Inflows:	Revenue: - Patient Services Revenue - Routine Check-ups - Cleanings - Dental Procedures - Other Patient Services - Other Revenue - Product Sales - Rental Income (if applicable) - Other Sources of Revenue Total Cash Inflows
Cash Outflows:	Cost of Goods Sold (COGS): - Dental Supplies - Lab Fees - Other Direct Costs Total Cost of Goods Sold Operating Expenses: - Rent - Utilities - Salaries and Benefits - Office Supplies - Marketing and Advertising - Equipment Maintenance - Professional Fees - Other Operating Expenses Total Operating Expenses Net Operating Income (NOI) Other Income and Expenses: - Interest Income - Investment Gains/Losses - Taxes - Depreciation - Amortization - Other Income/Expenses Total Other Income and Expenses Total Cash Outflows
Net Cash Flow:	= Cash Inflows - Cash Outflows

The Cashflow Statement

- **Balance Sheet:**

Purpose: The balance sheet provides a snapshot of the dental office's financial position at a specific point in time. It lists the practice's assets (e.g., cash, equipment, accounts receivable), liabilities (e.g., loans, accounts payable), and equity (e.g., owner's equity) and illustrates the relationship between these elements.

Importance: The balance sheet helps dental office managers assess the practice's financial health, liquidity, and solvency. It provides insights into the practice's assets and liabilities, its overall financial stability, and its ability to meet long-term financial obligations. By comparing balance sheets over time, managers can track changes in the practice's financial position and make informed decisions to support its growth and sustainability.

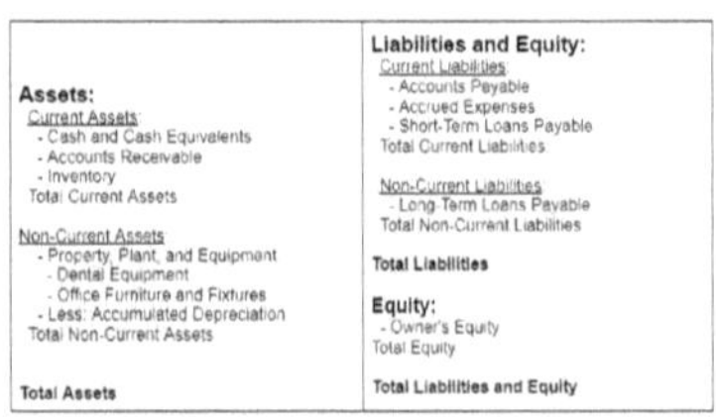

Assets:	**Liabilities and Equity:**
Current Assets: - Cash and Cash Equivalents - Accounts Receivable - Inventory Total Current Assets	Current Liabilities: - Accounts Payable - Accrued Expenses - Short-Term Loans Payable Total Current Liabilities
Non-Current Assets: - Property, Plant, and Equipment - Dental Equipment - Office Furniture and Fixtures - Less: Accumulated Depreciation Total Non-Current Assets	Non-Current Liabilities: - Long-Term Loans Payable Total Non-Current Liabilities
	Total Liabilities
	Equity: - Owner's Equity Total Equity
Total Assets	**Total Liabilities and Equity**

The Balance Sheet

Assets=Liabilities + Equity

In other words, assets represent everything that a company or individual owns that has value, including cash, investments, property, equipment, and other tangible and intangible assets. This total value is equal to the sum of liabilities and equity, which represent the sources of funding for those assets.

2. Securing Funding Options

Launching a dental practice is an exciting adventure, but financial realities can quickly become roadblocks. This chapter equips you with the knowledge to navigate the diverse landscape of funding options, ensuring your dream practice doesn't get stuck at the starting line.

The Traditional Trail: Bank Loans

The traditional trail of securing bank loans remains a reliable avenue for funding a startup. Banks offer competitive interest rates, flexible repayment terms, and various loan options tailored to meet the specific needs of dental practices. With a solid business plan and good credit history, dentists can access the capital necessary to cover startup costs such as equipment purchases, office lease agreements, and initial staffing expenses. Additionally, bank loans provide the benefit of establishing a relationship with a financial institution, which can offer additional banking services and support as the practice grows. While the loan application process may require thorough documentation and assessment of financial viability, the stability and credibility of bank financing make it an attractive option for many dental professionals embarking on their entrepreneurial journey.

What to look for when choosing a dental startup bank loan:

- **Interest Rate**: The interest rate is a critical factor in determining the overall cost of the loan. Look for a competitive interest rate that fits your budget and financial capabilities.
- **Loan Term**: The loan term refers to the length of time over which you'll repay the loan. Longer loan terms typically result in lower monthly payments but may incur more interest over time. Shorter loan terms usually have higher monthly payments but can save you money on interest in the long run.
- **Loan Amount**: Ensure that the bank is offering the amount of funding you need to establish or expand your dental office. Compare the loan amount with your budget and projected expenses to make sure it meets your requirements.
- **Fees and Charges**: Pay attention to any upfront fees, closing costs, or ongoing charges associated with the loan. Common fees may include origination fees, application fees, appraisal fees, and prepayment penalties. Understanding the total cost of borrowing is essential for making an informed decision.
- **Repayment Structure**: Evaluate the repayment structure offered by the bank. Determine whether the loan requires fixed monthly payments or if there's flexibility in repayment schedules. Some loans may offer graduated repayment plans or interest-only payments initially, which could be beneficial for managing cash flow.
- **Collateral Requirements**: Find out if the loan requires collateral, such as property or equipment, to secure the financing. Collateral may affect the terms and conditions of the loan, including the interest rate and loan amount.
- **Credit Requirements**: Understand the bank's credit requirements and determine whether you meet the criteria for approval. Your credit history and score may influence the interest rate and terms offered by the bank.

- **Loan Approval Time**: Consider the time it takes for the bank to process and approve your loan application. If you need financing quickly, choose a bank that offers expedited approval processes and efficient customer service.
- **Flexibility and Customization**: Look for a bank that offers flexibility in loan terms and customization options tailored to your specific needs. Flexibility in repayment schedules, loan terms, and payment structures can make it easier to manage your finances.
- **Customer Service and Support**: Evaluate the level of customer service and support provided by the bank. Choose a lender that is responsive, transparent, and committed to helping you throughout the loan process and beyond.
- **Reputation and Stability**: Research the bank's reputation and stability in the industry. Consider factors such as financial strength, customer reviews, and longevity in the market to ensure you're working with a reputable and reliable lender.
- **Additional Services**: Some banks may offer additional services or benefits, such as financial planning assistance, insurance products, or business advisory services. Assess whether these additional offerings align with your needs and add value to your overall banking relationship.

SBA Loans: Government-Backed Boost

When contemplating avenues for financing a dental startup, government-backed Small Business Administration (SBA) loans warrant serious consideration. These loans come with distinct advantages, including favorable terms, lower down payments, and the added appeal of government security. While SBA loans provide an enticing opportunity for funding, it's crucial to consider the complexities of the application process and potentially longer approval times. Despite these considerations, the stability and support offered by government-backed financing make SBA loans an attractive option for dental professionals looking to establish or expand their practices.

Private Investors & Partnerships: Partnering for Growth

Private investors and partnership arrangements offer alternative routes to funding a dental startup, presenting both unique advantages and considerations. Partnering with private investors can provide a substantial capital injection and, in some cases, strategic guidance for business growth. However, it's essential to weigh the potential drawbacks, such as surrendering an equity stake in the practice and the importance of establishing clear legal agreements to mitigate any future conflicts or misunderstandings.

Crowdfunding & Alternative Paths: Unleashing the Power of Many

In today's digital age, crowdfunding and alternative funding platforms present exciting opportunities for dental entrepreneurs to access capital and harness the power of community support. These avenues offer advantages such as tapping into diverse funding sources and engaging with a broader audience. However, it's essential to recognize the marketing efforts required to effectively promote a crowdfunding campaign and ensure compliance with regulations and platform rules to maintain credibility and trust among backers.

As you navigate the myriad funding options available, it's crucial to move beyond mere choices and focus on finding the strategic fit that aligns with your specific needs and goals. Match your funding requirements with available options, carefully analyzing loan amounts, interest rates, and repayment terms in light of your startup costs and financial objectives. Additionally, consider your personal risk tolerance and comfort level with potential equity loss or stringent repayment schedules. Ultimately, strive to align with partners and platforms that share your vision for the future success and growth of your dental practice.

Securing the right funding is the fuel that ignites your dream practice. By understanding the traditional and innovative options, carefully assessing your risk tolerance and financial goals, and learning from real-world success stories, you can chart a personalized funding roadmap. Remember, the journey to financial success in your dental practice starts with making informed decisions.

V

Location and Facility Setup

1. Unveiling Your Target Audience: Demographic Deep Dive

Launching a dental practice is an exciting venture, but choosing the right location is the cornerstone of your success. This chapter delves into the key factors and strategies to consider when selecting your ideal practice home. Think of it as building your foundation – a solid base attracts patients, fosters growth, and ensures your practice will thrive for years to come.

Begin by gaining insight into the audience you aim to serve. Perform a comprehensive demographic analysis of your targeted area, taking into account:

- **Age**: Identify if the community comprises established families, young professionals, seniors, or a diverse mix.

- **Income Levels**: Assess whether your pricing structure aligns with the local purchasing capacity.
- **Lifestyle Preferences**: Determine whether the community values convenience, aesthetics, or specialized services.

Your practice's vision plays a crucial role in decision-making. Consider how you envision your practice: Are you aiming to establish a Medicaid-based dental office? Look for areas with lower socioeconomic status. Interested in focusing on cosmetic dentistry and Invisalign? Target millennials, Gen Z, and professionals in tech and other white-collar industries. Want to specialize in implants? Target older populations. If you aspire to offer comprehensive dental services and build a strong community presence, seek areas where families own homes and are rooted in the community. By aligning your practice with the specific needs and demographics of your target audience, you'll not only connect with potential patients effectively but also carve out a unique position in a competitive market.

Mapping Out Your Competition: Navigating the Dental Landscape

When establishing a dental practice, it's essential to conduct a thorough analysis of the competitive landscape to make informed decisions and position your practice effectively. This involves more than just identifying the number of existing practices in your chosen location. You'll want to delve deeper into various aspects of your competitors' operations to gain a comprehensive understanding of the market dynamics.

Firstly, consider the **number of practices** in the area to determine whether the market is saturated with dental services or if there's room for new entrants. Assessing the density of practices can help you gauge the level of competition you'll face.

Secondly, evaluate the **services offered** by existing practices. Look for gaps or unmet needs in the market that you could potentially address with specialized or niche services. By identifying areas where competitors may be under-serving patients, you can tailor your offerings to meet those needs and differentiate your practice.

Lastly, analyze **patient demographics** to understand the composition of the local population and their dental care needs. Consider factors such as age, income levels, lifestyle preferences, and cultural diversity. This insight can help you identify opportunities to target specific patient segments that may be underserved or have unique dental care requirements.

By conducting a comprehensive analysis of the competition, you'll be better equipped to strategically position your practice and carve out a distinct niche in the market. This proactive approach can help you avoid direct competition with established rivals and maximize your chances of success in the competitive dental landscape.

Accessibility and Visibility: More Than Just a Pretty Door

The importance of location extends beyond demographics. Consider the following priorities:

- **Proximity to Residential Areas**: Prioritize convenience for patient visits and foster loyalty. Being close to residential areas ensures ease of access and encourages regular attendance.
- **Visibility and Signage**: Enhance visibility by positioning your practice along main roads with clear, inviting signage.

A prominent presence not only attracts new patients but also builds brand awareness within the community.

Keep in mind that prioritizing convenience fosters long-term relationships with your patients, enhancing satisfaction and retention.

Regulations and Standards: Ticking All the Boxes

Before finalizing the lease agreement, it's imperative to ensure full compliance with regulations and standards:

- **Zoning and Regulations**: Thoroughly verify that the chosen location is officially approved for dental use and aligns with local ordinances and zoning regulations. This step helps prevent any legal complications down the line.
- **Accessibility Standards**: Prioritize inclusivity by confirming that the space adheres to the Americans with Disabilities Act (ADA) requirements. Ensuring accessibility not only meets legal obligations but also accommodates a diverse range of patients.

Neglecting these compliance measures can result in delays and costly retrofits. Therefore, it's essential not to overlook this critical step in the process.

Laying the Groundwork: Infrastructure and Technology

Building the right environment is pivotal to realizing your vision:

- **Layout and Design**: Assess if the space aligns with your needs, including the desired number of operatories, waiting area, and administrative spaces. Prioritize patient flow and operational efficiency to optimize the experience for both patients and staff.

- **Technology Infrastructure**: Ensure the space is equipped with robust internet connectivity, sufficient phone lines, and the potential for integrating digital technologies. Investing in a future-proof setup enables seamless adaptation to evolving technological advancements.

It's crucial to recognize that a thoughtfully designed and well-equipped space not only enhances the patient experience but also streamlines workflow efficiency for your team.

Negotiating Your Home Away from Home: Lease Terms and Finances

Be savvy when negotiating your lease. Keep an eye for the following items:

- **Lease Term and Renewal Options**: Align the lease term with long-term business goals and secure favorable renewal options for stability. Ideally, you should be asking for a 10-year lease with another 10-year renewal option.
- **Rent and Escalation Clauses**: Negotiate competitive rent rates and clarify escalation clauses for rent increases.
- **Tenant Improvement Allowance (TI)**: Request funds to customize and improve the space to meet practice needs.
- **Space Configuration and Improvements**: Ensure the lease reflects agreed-upon space configuration and improvement allowances.
- **Operating Expenses and CAM Charges:** Define tenant responsibilities for paying operating expenses and negotiate caps on increases

- **Use and Exclusive Rights**: Specify permitted uses and negotiate exclusive rights to prevent nearby competition.
- **Assignment and Subleasing:** Clarify terms for assigning or subleasing space, including consent requirements. Make sure the terms allow you tell sell your office and transfer the lease.
- **Termination and Default Provisions**: Understand conditions for termination and negotiate favorable terms.
- **Indemnification and Liability**: Define responsibilities for property damage, injury, or other liabilities.
- **Renovation and Maintenance Obligations**: Clarify responsibilities for property maintenance, repairs, and renovations.
- **Lease Guarantees and Security Deposits**: Discuss guarantees and negotiate terms for adequate protection.
- **Ingress and Egress Rights**: Ensure clear provisions for access to the premises, including parking and entry points.
- **HVAC and Utility Services**: Specify tenant responsibilities for HVAC installation and utility maintenance and repairs.
- **Insurance Requirements**: Address liability and property insurance coverage requirements.
- **Quiet Enjoyment:** Include provisions for quiet enjoyment of the premises.
- **Subordination, Non-Disturbance, and Attornment (SNDA)**: Request an SNDA agreement to protect leasehold interests.
- **Environmental Compliance**: Verify compliance with environmental regulations and address any concerns.
- **Confidentiality and Non-Disclosure**: Protect sensitive information shared during negotiations.

- **Dispute Resolution**: Clarify procedures for resolving disputes or disagreements.
- **Compliance with ADA and Building Codes**: Ensure compliance with ADA and building codes for accessibility and safety.
- **Maintenance and Repairs**: Clarify responsibilities for routine maintenance, repairs, and replacements of building systems, fixtures, and equipment. Specify timelines for addressing maintenance issues and procedures for reporting and resolving maintenance requests.
- **Signage and Branding**: Negotiate provisions for installing exterior and interior signage to promote your practice and enhance visibility. Discuss branding guidelines to ensure consistency with your practice's image and identity.
- **Parking and Accessibility**: Address parking arrangements for patients and staff, including the number of designated parking spaces, accessibility requirements, and provisions for overflow parking. Ensure compliance with ADA requirements for accessible parking spaces and entryways.
- **Utilities and Services**: Define the allocation of utility costs and responsibilities for maintaining utility services such as water, electricity, gas, and sanitation. Discuss provisions for handling utility disruptions or emergencies.
- **Security and Safety**: Address security measures and safety protocols to protect the premises, equipment, and occupants. Discuss requirements for installing security systems, surveillance cameras, and access controls to prevent unauthorized entry and mitigate risks.
- **Exclusivity Clauses**: Negotiate exclusivity clauses that prevent the landlord from leasing space to competitors within the same property or nearby locations. Protect your practice's

market position and patient base by securing exclusive rights within the vicinity.

- **Relocation and Expansion Rights**: Consider provisions for relocating or expanding the practice within the same property or complex. Negotiate rights to first refusal or priority for available spaces that better suit your needs as the practice grows.
- **Leasehold Improvements**: Discuss ownership and rights to leasehold improvements made during the lease term. Clarify whether improvements become the property of the landlord or tenant at the end of the lease and any provisions for restoring the premises to its original condition.

Building for Tomorrow: Scalability and Future-Proofing

Consider the Future:

- **Scalability**: Select a location conducive to growth, enabling the addition of operatories or expansion of services as your practice evolves. Choose a space with the flexibility to accommodate future growth.
- **Lease Flexibility**: Negotiate lease terms that allow for adjustments to space requirements over time. Avoid restrictive terms that could impede your practice's expansion. Maintain the agility to adapt to changing needs.

By prioritizing foresight and flexibility, you lay the groundwork for sustained success and adaptability as your patient base grows and your practice evolves.

Selecting the ideal location for your dental practice is a multifaceted process that requires careful consideration of various factors.

By conducting demographic analysis, assessing accessibility, staying informed about regulations, planning infrastructure, and envisioning future growth, you can establish a strong foundation for success. This chapter aims to equip you with the knowledge and confidence needed to make informed decisions, laying the groundwork for a thriving dental practice that meets the needs of your community and fulfills your entrepreneurial aspirations. It's important to note that you won't be navigating this journey alone; having a broker and attorney on your team will provide invaluable support and guidance throughout the process.

2. Designing an Efficient Office Layout

Your dental office layout is like a well-orchestrated symphony. Each element - from patient flow to technology placement - needs to *harmoniously coexist* to create a smooth, efficient, and welcoming experience for both your team and your patients. This chapter serves as your conductor, guiding you through the key principles and considerations for designing a practice that sings with functionality, aesthetics, and positive vibes.

The Overture: Seamless Patient Flow and Reception Symphony

First Impressions Matter: Place the reception area strategically near the entrance, ensuring a clear and inviting pathway. Offer easy access to check-in systems and amenities like restrooms.

A Calming Movement: Design a comfortable waiting space with ergonomic furniture, calming colors, and natural light. Provide engaging entertainment options and informative materials to ease wait times.

The Flow Symphony: Map out patient movement from arrival to departure. Streamline the journey with clear signage, designated waiting areas for different procedures, and efficient patient flow between operatories.

The Heartbeat: Efficient Operatories and Treatment Spaces

Strategic Arrangement: Group operatories logically based on treatment type, ensuring easy access for both staff and patients. Consider proximity to sterilization areas and shared resources.

Conductor's Comfort: Prioritize ergonomics. Opt for adjustable chairs, proper lighting, and accessible equipment placement to keep your team performing their best.

A Symphony of Cleanliness: Designate a centralized sterilization area for optimal workflow and efficient infection control protocols. Include easily cleanable surfaces, hands-free dispensers, and proper ventilation.

The Backstage: Collaborative and Efficient Administrative Spaces

Streamlined Score: Organize administrative spaces for seamless communication and easy access to patient records and scheduling systems. Utilize technology to optimize workflow and communication.

Staff Harmony: Foster a positive work environment with dedicated break areas featuring comfortable seating and kitchen facilities. Create designated spaces for team meetings and collaboration.

Technology Integration: Conducting the Future

Strategic Placement: Seamlessly integrate technology into your layout. Ensure computer workstations, imaging equipment, and diagnostic tools are readily accessible without hindering patient care.

The Future Soundtrack: Design with flexibility in mind to accommodate future technological advancements. Incorporate adaptable spaces and infrastructure for easy tech integration.

A Patient-Centric Encore: Privacy and Comfort

Confidential Conversations: Dedicate private consultation spaces for discussing treatment plans and addressing concerns in a safe and serene environment.

Accommodating All Melodies: Ensure accessibility for patients with special needs. Include features like wider doorways, lowered countertops, and designated parking spaces. Provide sensory-calming areas for those with sensitivities.

Crafting the perfect dental office layout isn't just about aesthetics; it's about creating a symphony of efficiency, comfort, and patient-centric care. By considering the elements discussed here, you can design a space that not only elevates your practice's performance but also resonates with your patients, ensuring a harmonious experience for everyone. Remember, a well-designed layout is an investment in your practice's long-term success and patient satisfaction. Now, go forth and conduct your dental masterpiece!

3. Acquiring Necessary Equipment and Technology

In the grand orchestra of a successful dental practice, equipment and technology play a central role. They're the instruments that deliver high-quality care, ensure smooth operations, and create a harmonious experience for both you and your patients. This chapter serves as your conductor, guiding you through the key considerations and strategies for selecting the right tools and technology to equip your dental startup for a flourishing future.

Tuning Up: Core Equipment Needs and Budget Harmony

Start with the Score: Conduct a thorough assessment of your essential equipment needs. Consider the services you offer, your target patient population, and future growth plans. Dental chairs, sterilization equipment, and diagnostic tools are crucial starting points.

Balancing Quality and Cost: Don't fall victim to budget dissonance. While affordability is important, remember that high-quality equipment offers long-term benefits, minimizing maintenance costs and ensuring consistent performance. Analyze warranties, maintenance plans, and potential return on investment.

Digital Revolution: Integrating Technology for a Flawless Performance

Sharpen Your Diagnostic Vision: Explore digital imaging solutions like digital radiography and intraoral scanners. These technologies enhance diagnostic accuracy, streamline procedures, and impress patients with their modern touch.

Practice Management Symphony: Choose a robust software system that seamlessly integrates scheduling, billing, and patient records. Ensure user-friendliness for both you and your staff, fostering efficiency and eliminating unnecessary administrative burdens. Consider cloud-based options for accessibility and collaboration.

Ergonomics: Playing in Comfort Matters

Invest in Ergonomic Harmony: Don't let discomfort disrupt the performance. Opt for adjustable dental chairs and operatories that prioritize both practitioner and patient comfort. Proper back support, headrests, and lighting are key to minimizing strain and enhancing the clinical experience.

Technology Placement: A Seamless Flow: Strategically position equipment and technology for optimal accessibility and workflow. Ensure everything is within easy reach, minimizing unnecessary movement and maximizing efficiency.

Future-Proofing Your Practice: Adapting to the Technological Encore

Scalability and Upgradability: Don't get stuck in a technological dead end. Select equipment and software with the ability to adapt and grow with your practice. Opt for modular systems and open platforms that allow for seamless integration of future advancements.

Stay Ahead of the Curve: Don't be a one-hit wonder. Actively stay informed about emerging technologies in the dental field. Regularly evaluate your equipment and software to identify opportunities for improvement, keeping your practice at the forefront of innovation.

Vendor Collaboration: Building a Strong Supporting Cast

Find Your Reliable Crew: Conduct thorough research to identify reputable suppliers. Seek recommendations, read reviews, and compare options. Look for vendors with established track records, excellent customer service, and access to the latest products.

Negotiate with Confidence: Remember, you're the conductor! Negotiate favorable terms with suppliers, considering factors like warranty options, financing arrangements, and potential discounts for bulk purchases. Building strong relationships ensures ongoing support and access to the best solutions.

Regulatory Compliance: Playing by the Rules Ensures a Smooth Performance

Maintain Harmony with Regulations: Ensure all equipment and technology meet regulatory standards and comply with industry guidelines. This includes adherence to safety regulations, infection control measures, and data privacy requirements.

Train Your Orchestra: Invest in comprehensive training programs for your staff. Ensure they effectively operate and maintain the acquired equipment and software. Well-trained staff maximizes the value of your investments and contributes to a smooth workflow.

Equipping your dental practice with the right tools and technology is not just about acquiring equipment; it's about crafting a harmonious environment that fosters high-quality care, operational efficiency, and a positive experience for everyone involved. By carefully considering your needs, integrating technology strategically, and building strong partnerships, you can create a practice that plays a beautiful symphony of success for years to come. Remember, you are the conductor, and this chapter provides the tools to orchestrate a thriving performance. Take the stage and create your dental masterpiece!

VI

Marketing and Branding

1. Crafting a Unique Value Proposition

Standing Out from the Crowd: Crafting Your Dental Practice's Unique Voice

In the bustling world of dentistry, it's not enough to simply open your doors and wait for patients to flock in. You need a way to cut through the noise, establish your individuality, and capture the hearts (and teeth) of your ideal patients. This chapter equips you with the tools to do just that – crafting a **Unique Value Proposition (UVP)** that sets your dental practice apart and turns you into a magnet for the patients you're meant to serve.

Unveiling Your Inner Rockstar: Discovering What Makes You Shine

Before you can shout your unique melody from the rooftops, you need to understand what makes your tune special. This introspection involves:

- **Identifying your differentiating features**: Are you a haven for tech-savvy patients with the latest 3D scanners and laser treatments? Do you offer specialized services like pediatric dentistry or focus on anxiety-free experiences? Pinpoint what sets you apart from the competition.
- **Defining your core values**: Are you passionate about personalized care and building relationships with your patients? Do you prioritize affordability and accessibility? Understanding your values forms the foundation of your UVP and shapes the experience you offer.

Putting Yourself in Your Patients' Shoes: Understanding Their Needs and Desires

Remember, your UVP isn't a self-portrait; it's a love letter to your ideal patient. To write it effectively, you need to know what makes their hearts sing:

- **Embrace the patient-centric approach**: Conduct market research and gather feedback to understand their fears, anxieties, and desired outcomes. What keeps them up at night when it comes to dental care? How can you address their specific concerns?
- **Listen to the whispers**: Leverage patient feedback to identify areas where your practice excels, whether it's your gentle touch, flexible scheduling, or transparent communication. Highlight these strengths in your UVP.

From Whisper to Anthem: Crafting a Clear and Compelling Message

Now that you know your strengths and understand your audience, it's time to craft a message that resonates:

- **Clarity is key**: Ditch the jargon and speak directly to your ideal patient. Imagine you're explaining your practice to a friend over coffee. Keep it simple, concise, and easy to understand.
- **Benefits over features**: Don't just list services; focus on the positive outcomes. Instead of saying you offer free X-rays, explain how they help you provide personalized treatment plans for a healthier smile. Show, don't tell.

Consider your marketing approach as a canvas for setting yourself apart in the dental landscape. In a sea of $99 specials, adopting this technique aligns you with the masses, turning dentistry into a commodified service. This risks reducing clients/patients to choosing solely based on price, undermining the unique emotional journey that healthcare, especially dentistry, encompasses.

Dentistry isn't merely a transaction; it involves a spectrum of emotions, ranging from fear and anxiety to building self-esteem, addressing functional chewing habits, and shaping lifestyles. Your marketing campaign should transcend the generic and delve into the emotional nuances that make your dental practice stand out.

Craft a brand that is a true reflection of what makes you special. Rather than emphasizing discounted prices, highlight the quality and uniqueness of your work. Shift the focus from lowering prices to showcasing the value and expertise you bring to the table.

Ask yourself, "Aside from price, what sets me apart?" Is it your personalized patient care approach, cutting-edge technology, or a unique philosophy? Tailor your marketing efforts to spotlight these differentiators, creating a brand that resonates with the emotions and needs of your target audience.

Remember, a successful marketing strategy in dentistry isn't about blending in with the crowd; it's about standing out by embracing what makes your practice extraordinary.

Branding Harmony: Integrating Your UVP into Every Note

Your UVP isn't just a tagline; it's the melody that runs through everything you do:

- **Consistent across platforms**: From your website and social media to your brochures and office décor, ensure your UVP shines through. Every touchpoint should reinforce your unique identity and messaging.
- **Visual storytelling**: Images are powerful. Use visuals that align with your values and UVP. Whether it's showcasing your advanced technology or capturing the warm, welcoming atmosphere of your practice, let your visuals tell the story.

Spreading the Word: Engaging the Right Audience

The world needs to hear your unique dental tune! Leverage diverse marketing channels:

- **Digital domination**: Develop a strong online presence with a user-friendly website, engaging social media content, and targeted online advertising. Share patient testimonials and highlight your UVP across all platforms.
- **Community connection**: Don't underestimate the power of local engagement. Sponsor community events, partner with local businesses, and participate in relevant initiatives. Show

how your practice contributes to the community and aligns with its values.

Fine-Tuning Your Performance: Adapting and Evolving

The dental landscape is dynamic, so your UVP should be too:

- **Data-driven decisions**: Track your marketing efforts and analyze patient feedback. Use data to understand what resonates and what needs tweaking. Adapt your UVP and messaging based on insights.
- **Embrace feedback**: Encourage patient feedback through surveys, reviews, and open communication. Understand how they perceive your value proposition and use their insights to refine your messaging and enhance patient satisfaction.

Crafting a unique value proposition isn't just about words; it's about capturing the essence of your dental practice and sharing it with the world. By understanding your strengths, addressing patient needs, crafting a clear message, integrating it into your branding, and continuously adapting your approach, you can become the go-to dentist for your ideal patients.

2. Developing a Marketing Plan

In the competitive world of dentistry, where every smile whispers a story, attracting the right patients requires more than just a neon sign. You need a captivating melody, a marketing masterclass, to entice them and build a strong brand presence. This chapter guides you through the key notes and movements, helping you compose a marketing symphony tailored to your unique dental startup.

Setting the Rhythm: Defining Your Goals and Aligning with the Practice Harmony

Before striking the first chord, establish clear, measurable objectives. Whether it's a dazzling crescendo of new patient acquisition, a spotlight on specific services, or building brand awareness, these goals become the roadmap for your marketing journey. Remember, your marketing should perfectly harmonize with the overall business goals of your practice, ensuring every note contributes to the symphony of success.

Knowing Your Audience: Unveiling the Faces in the Crowd

Imagine your ideal patient - their needs, desires, and even online habits. Create detailed "patient personas" to understand who you're trying to reach. Go beyond demographics; explore their preferred music (digital or traditional marketing?), their dancing shoes (social media or local events?), and tailor your marketing message to make them jump to the beat.

Selecting the Instruments: Orchestrating Diverse Marketing Channels

The digital world offers a multitude of instruments - a professional website as your stage, SEO and social media as your lighting crew, and online ads as your dazzling effects. But don't forget the traditional band! Explore print media, community events, and direct mail to reach a wider audience. Remember, a balanced blend of digital and traditional channels creates a richer symphony.

Budget and Resource Allocation: Playing It Smart with Every Note

Your marketing budget is your melody, so allocate resources strategically. Consider the cost-effectiveness of each instrument and campaign. Track your return on investment (ROI) like a conductor analyzing sheet music, tweaking and adapting based on data to ensure every note resonates and maximizes impact.

Content Marketing: Educating Your Audience and Sharing Your Expertise

Become the orchestra's storyteller. Develop content that educates and engages your audience. Blog posts, articles, videos, and infographics become your educational repertoire, addressing common oral health concerns, showcasing your expertise, and highlighting your unique services. Don't forget patient testimonials and success stories - these are the powerful vocals that add authenticity and build trust.

Building Your Online Reputation: Managing the Reviews and Standing Ovations

In the digital age, reviews are your applause. Encourage satisfied patients to leave positive feedback on platforms like Google and Yelp. Respond to any negative feedback promptly and professionally, turning potential boos into standing ovations. Optimize your Google My Business profile – it's your online billboard, attracting patients with accurate information, high-quality visuals, and regular updates.

Promotions, Loyalty, and Referrals: Encores and Repeat Performances

Strategic promotions and discounts are like exciting solos, attracting new patients or highlighting specific services. But remember, it's not just about applause; ensure these offerings align with your overall goals and contribute to long-term practice growth. Loyalty programs and referral incentives become your encore, rewarding existing patients and encouraging repeat performances.

Monitoring and Adapting: The Continuous Performance Enhancement

Marketing is a dynamic dance, demanding constant monitoring and adaptation. Define key performance indicators (KPIs) as your performance metrics - website traffic, conversion rates, patient acquisition costs, and retention. Analyze this data regularly, adjust your instruments and tempo based on trends, and embrace innovative technologies and communication strategies to keep your marketing symphony fresh and relevant.

Your dental practice's marketing journey is not just about attracting patients; it's about crafting a unique and powerful symphony that resonates with your ideal audience. By understanding your audience, utilizing diverse marketing channels, effectively managing your resources, and continuously adapting to the changing landscape, you can create a marketing masterpiece that attracts the right patients, builds a strong brand, and ensures your practice flourishes in the competitive world of dentistry. Remember, you are the conductor, and this chapter provides the tools to compose your own dental symphony of success. Now, step onto the stage and let your unique melody play!

3. Building an Online Presence and Social Media Strategy

In the digital age, silence is not an option for your dental practice. You need a powerful online presence that resonates with your target audience, and a social media strategy as harmonious as Beethoven's Fifth. This chapter serves as your conductor's baton, guiding you through the keynotes of crafting a compelling online presence and harnessing the social media stage to engage your audience and attract new patients.

Building Your Digital Stage: Crafting a Professional Website

Think of your website as the grand performance hall where you welcome patients. Make it:

- **User-friendly**: Navigation should be effortless, loading times swift, and mobile responsiveness a guarantee.
- **Visually appealing**: High-quality images, a cohesive design, and a clear brand identity set the stage for a memorable experience.
- **Informative**: Showcase your expertise with engaging content, highlight your unique services, and include clear calls to action for appointments or contact.

Optimizing for Search Engine Applause: SEO Strategies

Imagine search engines as the critics guiding patients to your door. To earn their praise:

- **Conduct keyword research**: Identify the terms patients use to find your services and weave them naturally into your website content.

- **Embrace local SEO**: Claim your Google My Business listing, optimize for location-specific keywords, and encourage positive online reviews. Stay updated: SEO is a dynamic field. Track algorithm changes and adapt your strategies to ensure constant visibility.

Choosing Your Social Media Platforms: Where Does Your Audience Applaud?

Not all platforms are created equal. Identify where your target audience spends their time online:

- **Facebook**: For general engagement and community building.
- **Instagram and Tiktok**: For visually appealing content and showcasing your practice environment.
- **X**: For real-time updates, industry news, and connecting with dental professionals.
- **LinkedIn**: For showcasing your expertise and connecting with potential referral partners.

Composing Engaging Content: Sharing Your Expertise and Making Your Audience Smile

Fill your social media with content that informs, entertains, and resonates with your audience:

- **Educational content**: Share bite-sized oral health tips, explain procedures, and offer behind-the-scenes glimpses.
- **Visual content**: Captivating images, patient testimonials, and video demonstrations grab attention and increase engagement.

- **Interactive content**: Polls, quizzes, and contests spark conversations and foster a sense of community.

Social Media Advertising: Expanding Your Reach with Targeted Notes

Boost your audience and promote specific services or events with targeted social media ads.Remember:

- **Choose your demographics wisely**: Reach the patients who matter most with laser-focused targeting.
- **Stay informed about algorithms**: Adapt your strategies as platforms update their algorithms to ensure consistent visibility.
- **Track your results**: Measure the effectiveness of your campaigns and adjust your approach for optimal return on investment.

Fostering Patient Engagement and Building Your Online Orchestra

Interaction is key to building a loyal online community:

- **Respond promptly to comments and messages**: Show your patients you care about their feedback and questions.
- **Encourage positive reviews**: Satisfied patients are your best advocates. Prompt them to leave positive reviews on platforms like Google and Yelp.
- **Showcasing patient stories**: Share compelling patient experiences with their consent, humanizing your practice and building trust.

Listening to the Analytics: Fine-Tuning Your Performance

Every social media platform offers powerful analytics tools. Use them to:

- **Identify your most engaging content**: Replicate formats and topics that resonate with your audience.
- **Track reach and engagement**: Measure the impact of your efforts and adjust your strategy accordingly.
- **Stay informed about trends**: Discover what's working in the dental social media landscape and adapt your approach to stay relevant.

Online Reviews and Reputation Management: The Power of Positive Feedback

Your online reputation matters. Here's how to manage it:

- Proactively encourage positive reviews: Make it easy for satisfied patients to leave feedback on platforms like Google and Yelp.
- Address negative feedback professionally: Respond promptly and transparently, demonstrating your commitment to patient satisfaction.
- Use reputation management tools: Monitor your online presence and track sentiment to identify areas for improvement.

Integrating Your Online Symphony: Connecting with Patients Through Every Note

Make your online presence seamless for patients:

- **Offer online appointment scheduling**: Streamline the booking process and provide patients with convenience.

- **Share regular updates and announcements**: Keep your audience informed about events, promotions, and practice news.
- **Connect your social media to your website**: Ensure a consistent brand experience across all platforms.

Building a compelling online presence and implementing a thoughtful social media strategy are integral components of modern dental practice marketing. By crafting a professional website, optimizing for search engines, engaging with social media platforms, creating compelling content, leveraging social media advertising, fostering patient engagement, monitoring analytics, managing online reviews, and integrating online communication, you can establish a digital footprint that enhances patient awareness, trust, and loyalty.

VII

Staffing and Human Recourses

1. Hiring Qualified Personnel

In the intricate world of dentistry, where a healthy smile is a shared triumph, your practice thrives not just on your expertise, but on the collective synergy of your team. This chapter empowers you, the dental entrepreneur, to cultivate a dream team – a cohesive, qualified workforce that propels your startup towards success.

Laying the Foundation: Identifying Your Staffing Needs

Before embarking on your talent hunt, map your practice's needs meticulously:

- **Chart the Roles**: Clearly define the roles and responsibilities needed for seamless operation. Consider clinical and administrative positions, support staff, and potential for future expansion based on your practice's scope and projected growth.

Crafting the Call to Action: Compelling Job Descriptions

Imagine job descriptions as captivating trailers for your ideal team members. Each one should:

- **Clearly Outline Responsibilities**: Describe specific tasks, expectations, and required skills for each role. Be transparent about the challenges and rewards of the position.
- **Embrace Your Practice's Values**: Infuse the description with your unique work culture, mission, and commitment to professional development. Attract candidates who resonate with your vision.

Casting Your Net: Attracting Top-Tier Talent

Don't limit your talent pool to a single platform. Explore diverse avenues:

- Leverage online job boards, professional networks, and dental associations.
- Partner with local universities and community colleges for student recruitment.
- Participate in career fairs and industry events.
- Harness the power of social media to cultivate employer branding. Showcase your practice's culture, perks, and commitment to team growth.

Beyond Skills: Interviewing for Cultural Fit

Technical skills are crucial, but cultural fit is the magic ingredient. Design a structured interview process:

- Utilize a mix of behavioral, situational, and technical questions. Assess both skills and the candidate's alignment with your values and work environment.
- Involve key team members in the process. Their insights into team dynamics and expectations are invaluable for evaluating cultural fit.

Building a Mosaic: Prioritizing Diversity and Inclusion

A diverse team enriches your practice and enhances patient care:

- Implement inclusive hiring practices. Partner with diverse organizations, utilize inclusive language in job descriptions, and avoid potential biases in interviews.
- Cultivate a workplace culture that celebrates differences and encourages open communication. This fosters a sense of belonging and empowers team members to contribute their unique perspectives.

Sharpening Your Tools: Skills and Training Programs

Even the most qualified candidates benefit from ongoing development:

- Identify essential skills for each role, both technical and soft. Prioritize continual learning and adaptability.
- Invest in training programs, mentorship opportunities, and professional development workshops. Equipping your team with the latest knowledge elevates their performance and fosters their growth.

More Than Compensation: Creating Competitive Packages

Competitive salary and benefits are essential, but go beyond the basics:

- Research industry standards and offer attractive packages. Consider offering flexible benefits, wellness programs, and career advancement opportunities.
- Tailor packages to individual needs and roles. Recognize the unique value each team member brings and incentivize their ongoing dedication.

Due Diligence: Conducting Reference Checks and Background Screening

Thorough checks ensure both professional competence and patient safety:

- Conduct comprehensive reference checks with previous employers, colleagues, and educators. Verify qualifications, work ethic, and cultural fit.
- Implement background screening processes where necessary. Ensure compliance with legal requirements, especially for positions involving patient care or sensitive information.

Building a thriving dental practice is a collaborative effort, where each team member plays a vital role. By understanding your staffing needs, crafting compelling job descriptions, attracting top talent, prioritizing cultural fit, investing in skills and training, and offering competitive compensation packages, you can cultivate a dream team that propels your practice towards success. This chapter equips you with the knowledge and tools to create a workforce that is not just qualified, but truly passionate about contributing to your vision and delivering exceptional patient care. Remember, your team is your foundation, and investing in their growth is an investment in the future of your practice. Now, go forth and assemble your dream team, ready to bring smiles to your community and contribute to a thriving dental practice!

2. Establishing Employee Policies

In the vibrant world of dentistry, where healthy smiles flourish with teamwork, establishing clear and comprehensive employee policies is not just a legal requirement, but a cornerstone of building a thriving team culture. This chapter serves as your guide to crafting an employee handbook and developing policies that empower your workforce, foster a positive work environment, and ensure legal compliance for your dental startup.

Building the Foundation: An Employee Handbook with Purpose

Think of your employee handbook as the constitution of your practice, outlining the rights, responsibilities, and expectations shared by both you and your team. Remember:

- **Define the Purpose and Scope**: Clearly articulate the handbook's goals, ensuring it covers crucial topics like employment rules, benefits, professional conduct, and safety protocols.

- **Stay Legally Compliant**: Regularly review and update the handbook to reflect changes in local, state, and federal employment laws. This ensures both you and your employees are protected.

Setting Expectations: Policies for Employment Rules and Conduct

Clarity is key to fostering a smooth workflow and a positive team dynamic:

- **Work Hours and Scheduling**: Define standard work hours, scheduling procedures, and expectations for overtime or flexible work arrangements. Include clear guidelines for requesting time off and managing unexpected absences.
- **Code of Conduct**: Establish professional expectations, addressing issues like dress code, communication protocols, and interpersonal relationships among staff members. This fosters a respectful and productive work environment.

Investing in Your Team: Benefits and Compensation

Attract and retain top talent by offering competitive compensation and valuable benefits:

- **Compensation Structure**: Clearly outline salary structures, bonus opportunities, and any other forms of remuneration. Specify payment procedures to avoid misunderstandings.
- **Employee Benefits**: Detail all benefits offered, including health insurance, retirement plans, and any additional perks.

Provide eligibility criteria and enrollment information to ensure a smooth onboarding process.

Growth and Development: Fostering Your Team's Success

Empowering your team to grow is an investment in your practice's future:

- **Continuing Education**: Communicate your commitment to professional development by outlining continuing education opportunities, training programs, and career advancement pathways within the practice.
- **Performance Evaluation Process**: Detail how performance will be assessed, including the frequency of evaluations, criteria used, and potential outcomes. This helps employees understand expectations and identify areas for improvement.

Safety First: Creating a Healthy Work Environment

Ensure the well-being of your team and patients by prioritizing safety:

- **Occupational Safety Guidelines**: Establish procedures for maintaining a safe work environment, including emergency protocols, reporting hazards, and proper use of equipment.
- **Health and Wellness Programs**: Promote employee well-being with initiatives like mental health resources, stress management techniques, and programs that encourage a healthy work-life balance.

Building a Diverse and Inclusive Team

Embrace different perspectives and experiences to create a stronger practice:

- **Non-Discrimination Policies**: Clearly state your commitment to diversity, inclusion, and equal opportunity. Develop policies that prohibit discrimination based on any protected characteristic.
- **Handling Workplace Harassment**: Establish a zero-tolerance policy for harassment and outline clear procedures for reporting, investigating, and handling such incidents.

Protecting Privacy and Data Security

Building trust involves safeguarding confidential information:

- Patient Confidentiality: Emphasize the importance of HIPAA compliance and patient privacy. Provide clear guidelines on handling patient information and the consequences of privacy breaches.
- Data Security Protocols: Establish data security protocols to protect both patient and practice information. Outline expectations for responsible technology use and data encryption practices.

Handling Conflict and Grievances Constructively

Conflict can arise, but open communication is key to resolution:

- **Grievance Reporting Mechanisms**: Create a transparent process for employees to raise concerns or grievances.

Outline steps for reporting issues, conducting investigations, and ensuring fair resolutions.

- **Conflict Resolution Strategies**: Develop strategies for addressing conflicts among staff members. Encourage open communication, mediation, and other conflict resolution techniques to maintain a harmonious work environment.

Supporting Your Team Through Life Changes

Recognize and support your employees' personal needs:

- **FMLA and Other Leave Entitlements**: Provide information on family and medical leave entitlements as required by applicable laws. Clearly communicate eligibility criteria, application processes, and the duration of allowed leave.
- **Maternity and Paternity Leave**: Outline policies related to maternity and paternity leave, addressing any additional benefits or support offered during these significant life events.

3. Fostering a Positive Team Culture

In the vibrant world of dentistry, where smiles blossom through teamwork, fostering a positive and collaborative culture isn't just optional, it's essential. This chapter equips you, the dental entrepreneur, with the key strategies and principles to cultivate a work environment where collaboration, communication, and mutual support flourish, propelling your practice towards success.

Laying the Foundation: Shared Values and a Unified Vision

Before embarking on your cultural journey, solidify the bedrock:

- **Articulate Core Values**: Clearly define the core values that will guide your team's interactions and behaviors. These values, reflecting the practice's identity, become the compass for a positive culture.
- **Align with Mission**: Ensure these values seamlessly align with the practice's broader mission. Every team member's efforts should contribute to achieving the practice's overarching goals and vision.

Building Bridges: Fostering Open Communication

Communication is the lifeblood of any thriving team:

- **Encourage Transparency**: Cultivate an environment where open and honest dialogue is the norm. Provide avenues for anonymous feedback to address concerns without fear of judgment.
- **Regular Team Meetings**: Schedule frequent gatherings to share updates, discuss challenges, and celebrate successes. These meetings strengthen bonds, keep everyone informed, and offer opportunities for collaborative problem-solving.

Synergy in Action: Collaboration and Teamwork

Teamwork makes the dream work, and here's how to make it happen:

- **Collaborative Activities**: Organize team-building activities that go beyond mere fun. Opt for collaborative projects that showcase individual strengths and foster a sense of camaraderie.

- **Cross-Training Opportunities**: Invest in cross-training programs. By expanding skill sets, you not only enhance individual capabilities but also create a team that can seamlessly support each other.

Recognizing & Celebrating: Fueling Motivation and Morale

Appreciation goes a long way in building a thriving team:

- **Individual Contributions**: Regularly acknowledge and celebrate individual achievements, milestones, and positive behaviors. This reinforces a culture of appreciation and motivates future excellence.
- **Collective Success**: Celebrate team-based accomplishments together. Sharing the joy of reaching performance goals, completing projects, or receiving positive patient feedback strengthens team bonds and fosters a sense of shared purpose.

Cultivating Growth: A Commitment to Professional Development

Investing in your team is an investment in your practice's future:

- **Skill Enhancement**: Support personal and professional growth by providing opportunities for skill enhancement. Consider sponsoring continuing education courses, workshops, or certifications relevant to their roles.

- **Career Advancement:** Outline clear pathways for career progression within the practice. Offering growth opportunities increases retention, boosts morale, and encourages continuous improvement.

Beyond Work: Crafting a Positive Work Environment

A work environment that feels good fosters good work:

- **Work-Life Balance:** Encourage a healthy work-life balance. Implement policies that support flexible scheduling, offer time-off options, and promote wellness programs. A well-rested and balanced team is a more productive and engaged team.
- **Comfortable Workspace**: Design a workspace that's not just functional but also aesthetically pleasing. A thoughtfully designed environment contributes to a positive atmosphere, enhances productivity, and fosters a sense of belonging.

Navigating Challenges: Conflict Resolution and Support

Even the best teams face disagreements. Here's how to navigate them constructively:

- **Conflict Resolution Protocols**: Establish clear procedures for resolving conflicts promptly and constructively. Ensure designated channels exist to address disputes fairly and respectfully.
- **Mediation and Support:** Offer mediation services or provide access to external support resources for complex conflicts. A

proactive approach to conflict resolution prevents negativity from affecting the team's culture.

Feedback is the Gift that Keeps on Giving: Continuous Improvement

Embrace feedback as a tool for growth:

- **Regular Feedback**: Regularly solicit feedback from team members on various aspects of the practice, including processes, communication, and team dynamics. Act on constructive feedback to drive continuous improvement.
- **Responsiveness and Adaptability**: Demonstrate responsiveness to feedback by implementing necessary changes. This shows that the team's voice matters and reinforces a culture of learning and adaptation.

Celebrating Diversity: Inclusion is Key

A diverse team brings a wealth of perspectives, enriching your practice:

- **Inclusive Practices**: Foster an environment where everyone feels respected, heard, and valued, regardless of background or identity. Implement inclusive practices that embrace diversity in all its forms.
- **Diverse Perspectives**: Recognize and celebrate the unique perspectives and ideas each team member brings to the table. A diverse team fosters innovation, creativity, and problem-solving abilities.

Fostering a positive team culture is not only beneficial for the well-being of your team members but also crucial for the success of your dental practice. By defining team values, promoting open communication, encouraging collaboration, recognizing achievements, providing professional development opportunities, creating a positive work environment, resolving conflicts promptly, encouraging feedback, and emphasizing inclusivity, you can build a cohesive and resilient team that contributes to the overall success and reputation of your practice. This chapter serves as a guide for dental entrepreneurs seeking to create and sustain a positive team culture within their startup.

VIII

Patient Acquisition and Retention

1. Effective Patient Communication

In the world of dentistry, where smiles bloom from trust and understanding, effective patient communication isn't just a skill, it's the lifeblood of your practice. This chapter equips you, the dental entrepreneur, with strategies to forge meaningful connections with your patients, ensuring a positive and lasting experience that fuels growth and sustainability.

Laying the Foundation: Clear Communication Channels & Welcoming Reception

- **First Impressions Matter:** Train your front desk staff to embrace warmth and efficiency. Provide them with comprehensive information to confidently answer questions and guide patients through their interactions.

- **Communication Hubs**: Establish clear and accessible communication channels. Offer phone lines, email, a user-friendly website, and social media presence. Ensure patients can easily reach you for appointments, inquiries, or emergencies.

Trust Through Transparency: Building Bridges of Understanding

- **Treatment Clarity:** Break down the complexities. Clearly explain treatment plans, procedures, and associated costs. This empowers patients to make informed decisions about their oral health journey.
- **Empowering Education**: Offer educational materials that demystify common dental issues, preventive care, and the value of regular checkups. Informed patients become engaged partners in their health.

The Power of Empathy: Active Listening and Judgment-Free Zones

- **Patient-Centered Interactions**: Train practitioners to approach interactions with empathy and active listening. Understanding concerns, fears, and expectations fosters trust and comfort.
- **Creating a Safe Space**: Ensure patients feel comfortable discussing their oral health without fear of judgment. This open dialogue allows you to uncover underlying issues and address patient needs effectively.

Embracing Technology: Enhancing Accessibility and Convenience

- **Appointment Reminders**: Leverage modern tools. Implement SMS, email, or automated call reminders to reduce no-shows and keep patients informed about their visits.
- **Telehealth and Virtual Consultations:** Explore the potential of telehealth for virtual consultations or follow-ups. This technology enhances accessibility for patients with time constraints or transportation challenges.

Beyond Clinical Care: Personalizing the Patient Experience

- **Detailed Patient Profiles**: Maintain robust patient profiles and histories. This enables personalized care and meaningful conversations about each patient's unique oral health journey.
- **Personalized Touches:** Send birthday greetings, treatment anniversary reminders, or other personalized communications. These gestures strengthen the patient-practice relationship and demonstrate that you care.

Empowering Knowledge: Active Learning and Educational Resources

- **Interactive Sessions**: Organize workshops or in-house educational sessions. Cover topics like oral hygiene techniques, common dental issues, and Q&A sessions with practitioners.
- **Online Resource Hub:** Develop an online library of educational resources like articles, videos, and infographics on your website. This empowers patients to learn at their own pace and stay informed about their oral health.

Listening and Taking Action: Feedback as a Gift

- **Open Communication Channels:** Regularly solicit feedback through surveys, online forms, or in-person conversations. Analyze responses to identify areas for improvement and implement changes based on patient suggestions.
- **Responsiveness is Key:** Show you care by addressing patient concerns promptly and directly. This proactive approach demonstrates your commitment to patient satisfaction and fuels positive experiences.

Fostering Loyalty and Appreciation: Going Beyond Clinical Care

- **Loyalty Programs**: Implement loyalty programs where patients earn rewards for regular visits, referrals, or participation in preventive care programs. This incentivizes retention and builds stronger bonds.
- **Patient Appreciation Events**: Organize patient appreciation events or promotions to celebrate milestones, anniversaries, or special occasions. These initiatives create a sense of community and reinforce your commitment to your patients.

Setting Realistic Expectations: Clear Communication, No Surprises

- **Honesty is Best Policy**: Set realistic expectations about treatment outcomes, recovery times, and potential discomfort. Open communication about what patients can expect leads to greater satisfaction.
- **Proactive Approach**: Prevent misunderstandings about treatment plans or costs. Clearly communicate any potential variations and address patient concerns promptly.

Effective patient communication is not just a skill, it's the foundation of a thriving dental practice. By building trust through transparency, practicing empathy, utilizing technology, personalizing interactions, empowering knowledge, actively listening, fostering loyalty, and setting realistic expectations, you create a patient-centric environment that attracts, retains, and nurtures long-lasting relationships. This chapter serves as your guide to cultivate effective communication strategies and build a practice where smiles bloom not just from healthy teeth, but from genuine connections and trust. Remember, your patients are the heart of your success, and open communication is the key to unlocking their loyalty and satisfaction.

2. Creating a Patient-Centric Experience

In today's competitive dental landscape, simply offering good teeth cleanings isn't enough. To truly thrive, you need to prioritize a patient-centric experience, making every interaction feel personalized, comfortable, and focused on individual needs. This chapter equips you, the dental entrepreneur, with the strategies and principles to transform your startup into a haven of exceptional care, fostering patient satisfaction and loyalty that fuels your long-term success.

From Waiting Room to Wow Room: Crafting a Welcoming Atmosphere

- **Comfort is Key**: Design waiting areas that soothe nerves, not anxieties. Invest in ergonomic seating, calming décor, and soft lighting. Offer amenities like Wi-Fi, refreshments, and entertainment options for children.

- **Accessibility for All**: Ensure your practice is welcoming to everyone. Implement wheelchair accessibility, clear signage in multiple languages, and sensory-friendly accommodations for individuals with diverse needs.

Streamlining the Journey: Frictionless Appointment Management

- **Easy Booking**: Offer multiple appointment booking options, from online platforms to phone calls. Optimize systems for efficiency and flexibility, accommodating diverse schedules and minimizing wait times.
- **Tech-Powered Check-In:** Embrace digital check-in processes to reduce paperwork and administrative burdens. Let patients focus on their well-being, not forms, with user-friendly kiosks or mobile apps.

Beyond Check-Ups: Personalized Treatment Plans and Informed Decisions

- **Tailored Care:** Move away from one-size-fits-all approaches. Consider each patient's unique oral health history, lifestyle, and goals to craft personalized treatment plans that truly address their needs.
- **Empowering Conversations**: Clearly explain treatment options, potential benefits, risks, and costs. Use visual aids and open dialogue to empower patients to make informed decisions about their oral health journey.

Knowledge is Power: Cultivating Informed and Engaged Patients

Consultations with a Twist: Don't just examine teeth; educate! Utilize consultations to explain procedures, address questions, and provide educational materials that demystify oral health and treatment options.

Beyond the Visit: Implement ongoing patient education initiatives. Develop newsletters, workshops, or online resources to empower patients with knowledge and promote proactive oral care habits.

Communication is Key: Staying Connected and Building Trust

- **Proactive Reminders:** Utilize automated systems for appointment reminders and confirmations. Regular communication reduces no-shows and reinforces your commitment to patient care.
- **Follow-Up is Care:** Don't just treat, follow up! Initiate post-treatment phone calls or messages to check on patients' well-being. This demonstrates genuine concern and fosters a sense of ongoing support.

Technology as a Partner: Enhancing Care and Convenience

- **Digital Revolution:** Utilize digital records and imaging technologies to enhance diagnostic accuracy and share information seamlessly with patients. Visual aids contribute to better understanding and shared decision-making.
- **Telehealth Advantage**: Explore telehealth options for virtual consultations or follow-ups. This is especially beneficial for patients with mobility challenges or those seeking initial guidance before an in-person visit.

Listening and Learning: Embracing Feedback for Continuous Improvement

- **Open Feedback Channels**: Implement patient satisfaction surveys and feedback mechanisms through multiple channels. Actively seek input on their experiences to identify areas for improvement and celebrate successes.
- **Feedback into Action:** Don't just collect feedback, act on it! Demonstrate responsiveness by implementing improvements based on patient suggestions. This iterative process reinforces your commitment to continuous improvement.

Smooth Operations: Making Administrative Tasks Seamless

- **Billing Transparency**: Streamline billing and insurance processing to minimize administrative hassles for patients. Provide clear explanations of costs and assist them in navigating insurance claims.
- **Flexible Policies:** Craft patient-friendly policies for cancellations, rescheduling, and billing disputes. Flexibility and understanding contribute to a positive experience even in challenging situations.

Building Bridges: Community Outreach and Engagement

- **Local Health Champion**: Participate in community health initiatives to promote oral health awareness. Sponsor local events, provide educational sessions, and actively engage with the community to position your practice as a trusted partner in health.
- **Collaborative Care**: Forge partnerships with local organizations, schools, or businesses for collaborative health and wellness

programs. Community engagement not only benefits public health but also enhances your practice's reputation.

Creating a patient-centric experience is not just about providing good dental care; it's about building trust, fostering loyalty, and ensuring every patient feels valued and understood.

3. Loyalty Programs and Referral Systems

In the competitive world of dentistry, simply offering good teeth cleanings won't make you stand out. You need to create a community, a tribe of loyal patients who not only trust your expertise but also become your passionate advocates. This chapter equips you, the dental entrepreneur, with the strategies and principles to cultivate lasting relationships and ignite organic growth through impactful loyalty programs and referral systems.

Beyond Transactions: Building the Foundation of Loyalty

- **Understanding the Why**: Recognize that patient loyalty isn't just about discounts; it's about fostering personal connections and exceeding expectations. Loyal patients become your extended family, championing your practice and contributing to long-term sustainability.
- **The Impact Equation**: Remember, loyal patients equal recurring revenue and powerful word-of-mouth marketing. They provide invaluable stability and amplify your reach, attracting new patients who trust their network's recommendations.

Crafting Your Loyalty Program: It's All About Them

- **Tailored Rewards**: Don't offer a one-size-fits-all approach. Understand your patient demographics and preferences. Consider offering discounts, free services, exclusive events, or even priority scheduling to truly resonate with their needs.

- **Tiering for Growth**: Implement tiered systems that reward increased engagement. As patients progress, offer escalating benefits like bonus points, personalized consultations, or early access to new services, incentivizing their continued loyalty.

Technology as Your Partner: Streamlining and Insights

- **Digital Platforms:** Explore user-friendly platforms to seamlessly track patient engagement and reward distribution. Automate processes, track visits, and gain valuable insights into patient behavior to refine your program.

- **Integrated Power**: Integrate your loyalty program with your practice management system. This ensures accurate tracking, efficient reward distribution, and a smoother experience for both you and your patients.

Communicating Value: Making Loyalty Irresistible

- **Clear and Consistent:** Effectively communicate the program's benefits through multiple channels, from your website and social media to in-practice signage and email newsletters. Ensure patients understand the value proposition and how to participate.

- **Educational Materials**: Create informative resources explaining the program's mechanics and highlighting the tangible benefits. This transparency builds trust and encourages active engagement.

Unleashing the Power of Referrals: Friends Bring Friends

- **Recognize the Ripple Effect**: Acknowledge the immense impact patient referrals can have. They bring new faces to your practice, fueled by the positive experiences of existing patients, creating a powerful cycle of growth.
- **Incentivize and Reward:** Consider offering attractive rewards within your loyalty program specifically for referrals. This mutual benefit system motivates patients to advocate for you and expands your reach exponentially.

Word-of-Mouth Marketing: Making Them Your Ambassadors

- **Create Shareable Experiences:** Make every visit positive and memorable, encouraging patients to share their experiences online through reviews, social media posts, or personal recommendations.
- **Empower Them with Content**: Craft engaging content – informative articles, patient testimonials, or fun promotional materials – that patients can easily share with their networks, amplifying your reach and visibility.

Social Media: The Engagement Hub

- **Engage Loyally:** Leverage social media to interact with loyalty program participants. Share program updates, recognize member achievements, and create a sense of community that fosters deeper loyalty and connection.
- **Promote Referrals:** Use your social media platforms to highlight your referral program. Encourage patients to share their experiences and incentivize them to refer friends and family, extending your reach organically.

Data-Driven Decisions: Measuring and Adapting

- **Track and Analyze**: Don't operate in the dark. Use data analytics to track the performance of your loyalty program and referral initiatives. Analyze participation rates, redemption rates, and referral campaign success to identify areas for improvement.
- **Adapting for Growth**: Utilize the insights from your data to refine your strategies. Address challenges, capitalize on successful aspects, and continuously optimize your loyalty and referral systems for maximum effectiveness.

Showcasing Success Stories: Celebrating Loyalty

- **Highlight Beneficiaries**: Share stories of patients who have thrived through your program. Showcase how their loyalty has yielded positive outcomes like improved oral health, access to exclusive services, or even community engagement.
- **Inspire Others**: These real-life examples demonstrate the program's value and inspire other patients to participate, strengthening your community and fueling further growth.

Effective loyalty programs and referral systems are not just marketing tools; they are the seeds you plant to cultivate a thriving community of loyal patients who become your biggest advocates. By understanding the power of loyalty, designing engaging programs, leveraging

IX

Technology Integration

1. Implementing Dental Management Software

In today's dynamic dental landscape, technology isn't just a perk, it's a necessity. Dental Management Software (DMS) stands at the forefront, transforming practices into efficient, patient-centric hubs. This chapter empowers you, the dental entrepreneur, to navigate the world of DMS, from selection to seamless implementation, unlocking its potential to elevate your practice and delight your patients.

Unveiling the Powerhouse: The Role of DMS

Imagine a central hub seamlessly managing your entire practice - patient records, appointments, finances, and more. That's the magic of DMS. It streamlines operations, boosts accuracy, and frees your team to focus on what matters most: exceptional patient care.

Finding Your Perfect Fit: Tailoring DMS to Your Needs

Before diving in, take a deep breath and assess your practice. How many patients do you see? What services do you offer? What workflows do you use? These answers guide your DMS selection, ensuring it complements your unique setup and fuels smooth scaling.

Exploring the Treasure Chest: Key Features That Matter

Now, let's explore the treasure chest of DMS features:

- Patient Records & Scheduling: Ensure robust tools for patient information management and appointment scheduling. Think user-friendly interfaces, intuitive data entry, and seamless access to medical histories.
- Billing & Financial Management: Say goodbye to administrative headaches! Look for features like automated invoicing, insurance claim processing, and comprehensive financial reports. Streamlined finances mean more time for growth.
- Imaging & Diagnostics: Level up your diagnostics with DMS that integrates seamlessly with imaging and diagnostic tools. Think efficient storage, instant data retrieval, and a cohesive approach to patient care.

Building Bridges: Enhancing Patient Communication

Communication is key to thriving relationships. Choose a DMS that facilitates it flawlessly. Imagine automated appointment reminders, follow-up messages, and even patient portals for online access to records and educational materials. Happy, informed patients become loyal advocates.

Empowering Your Team: Training and Support Are Crucial

Prioritize comprehensive training for your team to master the DMS. Think immersive programs, ongoing support, and readily available technical assistance. Remember, empowered staff equals a thriving practice.

Security First: Protecting Your Data and Peace of Mind

Patient data is sacred. Choose a DMS that prioritizes HIPAA compliance and robust security measures. Regular audits, secure data storage, and access control protocols are non-negotiable for peace of mind.

Adaptability is Key: Evolving with Technology

The dental world is dynamic, and your DMS should be too. Opt for a system that allows customization to match your evolving workflows and integrates seamlessly with emerging technologies. Remember, flexibility is the name of the game.

Beyond the Migration: Navigating Data Seamlessly

Transitioning to a new DMS can be daunting, but planning makes it smooth. Conduct thorough data audits, ensure data accuracy, and establish secure protocols for transferring patient records. Data migration done right paves the way for success.

Your Practice, Transformed: Embracing the Future

Implementing DMS is a transformative step. By understanding its role, assessing your needs, exploring key features, integrating with technology, prioritizing communication, empowering your team, ensuring security, embracing adaptability, navigating data migration, and learning from success stories, you'll unlock a world of efficiency, patient-centric care, and practice growth. With DMS as your partner, your dental startup is poised to revolutionize the way you deliver exceptional care and build a thriving community of loyal patients. Remember, the future of dentistry is digital, and you hold the key to unlocking its potential.

2. Incorporating Telehealth and Virtual Consultations

In today's tech-driven world, patients expect flexibility and convenience. Telehealth and virtual consultations are no longer a novelty, but a crucial component of a modern dental practice. This chapter empowers you, the dental entrepreneur, to harness the power of telehealth, seamlessly integrating it into your startup to expand accessibility, enhance patient experience, and revolutionize the way you deliver care.

Beyond Distance: The Power of Telehealth in Dentistry

Imagine patients in remote areas accessing expert consultations, busy professionals scheduling appointments from their desks, and anxious individuals receiving guidance from the comfort of their homes. Telehealth bridges geographical barriers, promotes convenient and flexible care, and ultimately, makes quality dental services accessible to all.

Tailoring Telehealth to Your Dentistry Expertise

Not all consultations are created equal. While comprehensive oral examinations require in-person presence, telehealth shines in various specialty areas:

- **Preventive Care**: Discuss oral hygiene techniques, dietary habits, and lifestyle factors impacting oral health remotely.
- **Initial Consultations**: Provide initial assessments, discuss treatment options, and address patient concerns virtually.
- **Post-Treatment Follow-Ups**: Monitor progress, answer questions, and offer ongoing support without requiring physical visits.

Choosing Your Toolkit: User-Friendly Platforms and Seamless Integration

Navigating technology shouldn't be a chore. Choose user-friendly telehealth platforms that:

- **Prioritize user experience**: Easy for both you and your patients to navigate, ensuring a smooth virtual interaction.
- **Comply with regulations**: Adhere to healthcare privacy and security standards like HIPAA to protect patient data.
- **Integrate seamlessly:** Integrate with your existing practice management system for streamlined scheduling, recordkeeping, and billing.

From Protocol to Practice: Establishing a Telehealth Framework

Clear guidelines are crucial for success. Define protocols for:

- **Scheduling appointments**: Ensure a smooth virtual booking process for both parties.

- **Conducting secure video calls**: Utilize HIPAA-compliant platforms and maintain professional conduct during consultations.
- **Documenting virtual interactions**: Clearly document key details of virtual consultations for accurate patient records.
- **Handling emergencies**: Outline procedures for urgent situations that may arise during virtual appointments.

Spreading the Word: Educating and Engaging Your Patients

Don't keep telehealth a secret! Inform your patients about this convenient option:

- **Utilize various channels**: Announce it on your website, social media, email newsletters, and even in-practice signage.
- **Highlight benefits**: Emphasize reduced travel time, increased flexibility, and timely access to care.
- **Educate on how it works**: Explain the process, technology used, and potential benefits for their specific needs.

Beyond Consultations: Integrating Telehealth into Treatment Plans

Telehealth isn't just for initial visits. Consider incorporating it into your treatment plans:

- **Virtual follow-ups:** Monitor progress, address concerns, and provide ongoing support post-treatment remotely.

- **Preventive care reminders and education**: Offer virtual sessions to reinforce proper oral hygiene and answer questions.
- **Remote monitoring of certain conditions**: Utilize specific technologies for certain cases, allowing patients to track progress from home.

Navigating the Regulatory Landscape: Compliance is Key

Protecting patient data and adhering to regulations are paramount. Ensure:

- **HIPAA compliance**: Implement robust safeguards to protect patient confidentiality and data security.
- **Awareness of evolving regulations**: Stay updated on changing telehealth regulations and adapt your practices accordingly.

Empowering Your Team: Training for Seamless Telehealth Delivery

Your team is your telehealth ambassador. Invest in training to:

- **Master the technology**: Ensure staff members are proficient in using the chosen platform and troubleshooting any issues.
- **Develop effective communication skills**: Train them to build rapport, actively listen, and address patient concerns effectively remotely.

- **Embrace a telehealth mindset:** Foster a team culture that values the role of virtual consultations in enhancing patient care.

Making it Clear: Transparent Fee Structures and Insurance Considerations

Finances shouldn't be a barrier. Be transparent about fees:

- **Clearly communicate costs**: Inform patients about the costs associated with virtual consultations and any related services.
- **Understand insurance coverage**: Stay informed about insurance coverage and reimbursement policies for telehealth services.
- **Guide patients through reimbursement**: Assist patients in understanding and accessing insurance reimbursements for telehealth.

3. Staying Updated with Dental Technology Advancements

The AI Revolution in Dentistry: Empowering Your Startup for Growth and Innovation

The tide is turning in dentistry. Gone are the days of static practices clinging to traditional methods. Now, a wave of technological advancements, spearheaded by Artificial Intelligence (AI), is transforming the landscape, and dental startups are poised to ride the crest. This chapter serves as your navigational compass, charting the course towards integrating AI into your practice, optimizing workflows, and ultimately empowering your startup for growth and innovation.

Embracing the Digital Wave: Where Dentistry Meets Technology

Imagine a world where patient records seamlessly flow between systems, AI assistants handle routine inquiries, and diagnostics are revolutionized by intelligent algorithms. This isn't science fiction; it's the reality of digital dentistry. By embracing this shift, you unlock a world of possibilities for your patients and practice.

AI-Powered Diagnostics: Seeing Beyond the X-ray

Dental radiographs are crucial, but AI takes image analysis to the next level. Imagine algorithms detecting subtle anomalies invisible to the human eye, aiding in early-stage disease detection and facilitating more precise treatment plans. This is the power of AI in diagnostics, and it's changing the game.

Scheduling that Works Smarter, Not Harder

Say goodbye to appointment woes! AI-powered scheduling systems analyze historical data, patient preferences, and practitioner availability to create a personalized and efficient schedule. No more missed slots or patient frustration – just a smoothly flowing calendar that boosts your productivity.

Communication Elevated: From Robots to Rapport

AI isn't replacing your empathetic touch; it's amplifying it. AI-powered systems can handle routine inquiries, freeing up your team for complex interactions. Imagine chatbots answering basic questions, sending appointment reminders, and even analyzing phone calls to identify areas for communication improvement.

AI's Expanding Portfolio: A Glimpse into the Future

This is just the beginning. Imagine AI personalized treatment plans, predictive models for caries risk, and chatbots offering educational resources tailored to each patient's needs. The potential of AI in dentistry is vast, and staying ahead of the curve is key to future success.

Adapting to the AI Age: Embracing Transformation, Not Fearing Disruption

Change can be daunting, but with the right approach, it becomes an opportunity. Foster a culture of continuous learning within your team, encouraging them to embrace AI and become advocates for its integration. Invest in training, workshops, and collaborations with tech providers to ensure a smooth transition.

Ethics at the Forefront: Balancing Innovation with Responsibility

As AI takes center stage, ethical considerations must be paramount. Prioritize patient privacy and data security. Implement robust measures to protect information and ensure transparency in how AI algorithms are used. Remember, ethical practice is the foundation of successful innovation.

Collaboration is Key: Partnering for Progress

Don't go it alone! Forge partnerships with tech providers specializing in dental AI solutions. These collaborations offer access to cutting-edge technology, ongoing support, and valuable insights into the ever-evolving landscape. Additionally, consider partnering with research institutions to contribute to advancing AI in dentistry and shape the future of the field.

Efficiency Unleashed: AI's Impact on Your Practice

By leveraging AI, you can significantly boost your practice's efficiency. Imagine automated tasks, streamlined workflows, and faster diagnostics – all freeing up your team to focus on what matters most: delivering exceptional patient care.

More Than Efficiency: Enhanced Patient Experience, Elevated Satisfaction

The benefits go beyond numbers. AI offers patients a more personalized and convenient experience, from automated reminders to virtual consultations. Imagine reducing wait times, providing targeted educational resources, and fostering a sense of empowered participation in their oral health journey. This, in turn, translates to increased patient satisfaction and loyalty.

The AI revolution in dentistry is here, and its impact is undeniable. By embracing this transformative technology, you can position your startup as a leader in innovation, optimize your practice efficiency, and ultimately, deliver exceptional, patient-centric care. Remember, the future of dentistry is intelligent, adaptable, and most importantly, centered on empowering both patients and practitioners. This chapter equips you with the knowledge and insights to navigate this exciting new era and ensure your startup thrives in the AI-powered landscape of dentistry.

X

Financial Management

1. Implementing Accounting Systems

The heartbeat of any thriving dental practice is a solid financial foundation. This chapter empowers you, the dental entrepreneur, to navigate the essential world of accounting systems, transforming financial management from a daunting task to a strategic tool for growth and success.

From Numbers to Insights: Why Robust Accounting Matters

Imagine financial decisions fueled by crystal-clear insights, not guesswork. Robust accounting systems illuminate your practice's financial health, empowering you to make informed choices that align with your growth goals. Beyond strategic decision-making, they ensure you meet regulatory requirements and maintain transparency, both crucial for ethical and legal practice management.

Finding the Perfect Fit: Choosing Your Accounting Software

Every practice is unique, and your accounting software should be too. Start by identifying your needs: practice size, transaction volume, and specific features required. Prioritize user-friendliness; remember, efficient software empowers both practitioners and staff, minimizing training burdens.

The Powerhouse Features: What Your Software Needs

Imagine effortlessly tracking invoices, expenses, and cash flow. Choose software equipped with robust tracking features, ensuring meticulous bookkeeping and simplifying financial oversight. Integration with your existing practice management system is key for seamless data flow, minimizing errors and inconsistencies.

Tailoring Your Financial Map: The Chart of Accounts

Think of your chart of accounts as a customized financial map, reflecting your practice's unique revenue streams, expenses, and activities. Categorize and subcategorize to accurately track income, expenses, and identify areas for further analysis and informed decision-making.

Building Strong Habits: Streamlining Your Bookkeeping

Consistent data entry is paramount. Develop clear protocols for prompt recording of transactions, minimizing inaccuracies and offering real-time financial visibility. Regularly reconcile bank statements, invoices, and other documents to identify discrepancies and maintain data integrity.

Charting Your Course: Budgeting and Financial Planning

Develop realistic, goal-oriented budgets that consider short-term needs and long-term aspirations. Account for potential fluctuations in revenue and expenses, creating a roadmap for informed resource allocation. Regularly monitor your budget's performance against actual results, adapting as needed to capitalize on opportunities and navigate challenges.

Beyond Numbers: Financial Reporting and Analysis

Utilize your accounting software to generate comprehensive reports, including income statements, balance sheets, and cash flow statements. These offer a holistic view of your financial health. Go beyond traditional metrics; identify and analyze Key Performance Indicators (KPIs) specific to dentistry, such as patient retention rates and overhead costs, gaining valuable insights into operational efficiency and profitability.

Safeguarding Your Fort: Internal Controls and Security

Minimize financial risks by implementing internal controls. Distribute financial responsibilities across team members, ensuring proper oversight and minimizing the risk of errors or fraud. Implement robust audit trails and security measures to protect data integrity and confidentiality.

Navigating the Tax Maze: Planning and Compliance

Taxes are inevitable, but with proactive planning, they can be optimized. Leverage your accounting system to track deductible expenses, identify tax-saving opportunities, and ensure compliance with applicable tax laws. Collaborate with tax professionals for expert guidance, utilizing your accounting software to facilitate seamless communication and data sharing for accurate and efficient tax preparation.

Implementing effective accounting systems isn't just about managing numbers; it's about building a resilient financial fortress for your dental startup. By choosing the right software, customizing your financial map, establishing efficient bookkeeping practices, and prioritizing budgeting, reporting, internal controls, tax planning, and continuous learning, you create a foundation for sustained growth and fiscal prosperity. Let this chapter be your guide to navigating the financial landscape with confidence, transforming numbers into powerful tools for strategic decision-making and long-term success. Remember, in the world of dentistry, financial health is not just a number; it's the cornerstone of a thriving practice and a satisfied patient community.

2. Monitoring Key Performance Indicators (KPIs)

Imagine being able to peer into the inner workings of your dental practice, not just seeing numbers but gaining true understanding. Key Performance Indicators (KPIs) are the magic key that unlocks this hidden world, empowering you to make informed decisions, identify areas for improvement, and ultimately fuel the growth and efficiency of your dental startup.

KPIs: The Roadmap to Success

Think of KPIs as the strategic roadmap to your practice's success. They provide invaluable quantitative insights into various aspects, from patient acquisition to financial health. By monitoring these indicators consistently, you'll gain the clarity needed to align your strategies with overarching goals and continuously strive for improvement.

Finding the Right Compass: Selecting Relevant KPIs

Choosing the right KPIs is like picking the perfect instrument for the job. Consider focusing on areas crucial to your practice's success, such as:

- **Patient Acquisition and Retention**: Track new patient registrations, retention rates, and referral program effectiveness to understand patient flow and loyalty.
- **Appointment Scheduling and Utilization**: Monitor booked appointments, cancellations, and operatories use to optimize scheduling and resource allocation.
- **Financial Health**: Keep an eye on revenue growth, overhead costs, and profit margins to ensure financial stability and sustainability.

Operational Efficiency: Streamlining Your Practice

Dig deeper into your practice's efficiency:

- **Average Treatment Time**: Measure the average time per patient to identify areas for streamlining procedures and optimizing scheduling.
- **Operatory Turnover Rate**: Track how efficiently operatories are utilized. A high turnover rate often indicates efficient resource allocation.

Patient Satisfaction: The Heart of Your Practice

Your patients' happiness is key to success. Consider:

- **Net Promoter Score (NPS)**: This metric gauges patient loyalty and advocacy. A high NPS signifies satisfied patients who are more likely to recommend your practice.
- **Online Reviews and Ratings**: Monitor online feedback to understand patient experience and leverage positive reviews to attract new patients.

Marketing and Outreach: Measuring Your Impact

Track the effectiveness of your marketing efforts:

- **Conversion Rates from Marketing Campaigns**: Analyze how many leads convert into actual patients to understand which marketing strategies are most impactful.
- **Digital Engagement Metrics**: Monitor website traffic, social media interactions, and online appointment requests to assess the effectiveness of your online presence.

Beyond Numbers: Staff Productivity and Satisfaction

A happy and productive team is crucial:

- **Staff Turnover Rates**: Monitor turnover rates to identify potential issues affecting employee satisfaction and practice stability.
- **Productivity per Staff Member**: Measure individual productivity to optimize staffing and identify areas where additional support might be needed.

Embracing Technology: Measuring Tech's Impact

Track how technology is transforming your practice:

- Utilization of Dental Technology: Monitor the adoption and utilization of new technologies like digital x-rays, electronic health records, or telehealth services to assess their impact on patient care and efficiency.
- Training Completion Rates: Ensure your team is proficient in utilizing new technologies by monitoring training completion rates.

Compliance and Risk Management: Staying on Top

Proactive risk management is key:

- **Adherence to Regulatory Standards**: Track compliance with licensing requirements, infection control protocols, and data security measures to mitigate potential risks.
- **Incident Reporting and Resolution**: Monitor incident reporting and resolution rates to identify and address potential issues promptly.

Building Your KPI Dashboard: Visualizing Success

Imagine having a centralized hub for all your key metrics – a KPI dashboard. This visual representation allows for quick assessments, insightful comparisons, and data-driven decision-making.

Reporting and Analysis: Making Insights Actionable

KPIs alone tell just part of the story. Implementing regular reporting and analysis is crucial:

- **Schedule regular reviews**: Establish a cadence for reviewing your KPI dashboard and conducting deeper analyses to identify trends, strengths, and weaknesses.
- **Translate insights into action**: Don't let data collect dust! Use insights to drive strategic initiatives, optimize operations, and continuously improve your practice.

2. Planning for Long-Term Financial Success

Financial stability may not be the most glamorous aspect of running a dental practice, but it's the anchor that keeps you afloat, navigating the ever-changing tides of the healthcare landscape. This chapter delves into the depths of long-term financial planning, equipping you with the knowledge and tools to chart a course towards sustained growth and prosperity for your dental startup.

Setting sail with clear objectives:

Before embarking on your financial voyage, define your destination. Establish clear, quantifiable long-term goals that align with your overall vision. Do you aim to double your annual revenue within five years? Attract 20% more patients per month? Expand your practice to accommodate additional services? Having tangible targets guides your decision-making and provides benchmarks for measuring progress.

Weathering the storms with strategic planning:

Think beyond sunny skies. Develop a comprehensive financial plan that spans multiple years, incorporating budgeting, forecasting, and scenario analysis. Anticipate potential challenges like economic downturns or unexpected expenses, creating strategies to navigate them with minimal turbulence. Remember, adaptability is key to overcoming unforeseen storms.

Investing in growth, diversifying your treasure chest:

Reinvesting profits back into your practice is like reinvesting in your ship's sails. Consider upgrading equipment, expanding facilities, or incorporating advanced technologies like digital x-rays or CAD/CAM systems. This not only enhances patient care and operational efficiency but also attracts new patients and fuels growth.

However, don't put all your eggs in one basket. Explore diversification strategies beyond the practice itself. Real estate, stocks, or other investments can spread your risk and provide long-term financial security.

Building a resilient vessel: securing the hull and preparing for rough seas:

Establish an emergency fund as your life raft, weathering unforeseen economic storms. This buffer allows you to handle unexpected challenges without compromising the stability of your practice. Additionally, manage and strategically reduce existing debt, freeing up resources for investments and long-term financial health.

Planning for smooth transitions: ensuring your legacy lives on:

Your journey doesn't end with you. Incorporate succession planning into your strategy. Whether you envision bringing in new partners, selling the practice, or passing it on to the next generation, plan for a smooth transition that ensures the continued success of your legacy.

Continuous learning: keeping your compass calibrated:

Investing in the professional development of yourself and your team is like updating your navigational charts. Stay abreast of advancements in dentistry, business management, and technology to remain competitive and deliver high-quality patient care. Remember, the healthcare landscape is dynamic, and continuous adaptation is crucial for success.

Securing your personal horizon: charting a course for retirement:

Don't forget your own future. Prioritize retirement planning as part of your long-term strategy. Establish a savings plan through IRAs, 401(k)s, or other suitable investments. Seek professional advice from financial advisors specializing in healthcare professionals to optimize your retirement savings and plan for tax implications.

Building bridges with your community: anchoring your reputation:

Invest in community engagement. Sponsor local events, support local causes, or initiate outreach programs. Building a positive reputation fosters patient loyalty, referrals, and contributes to the practice's long-term sustainability. Remember, a strong community connection acts as an anchor, securing your position in the local landscape.

Embracing the digital wave: navigating technological currents:

The winds of technological change are constantly blowing. Stay informed about emerging trends like artificial intelligence, tele-dentistry, and digital treatment planning. Assess their relevance to your practice goals and plan for their integration to offer cutting-edge care and remain competitive. Remember, technology can be a powerful tool for driving efficiency and enhancing patient experience.

The voyage never ends: adjusting your sails for changing tides:

Regularly review your financial goals and strategies. Are you on track? Have market conditions or industry trends shifted? Be flexible and adapt your plan as needed. Remember, the journey towards financial success is an ongoing process, requiring constant evaluation and adjustments based on the ever-changing currents of the healthcare landscape.

Long-term financial planning is a compass guiding you towards financial security and sustainability. By setting clear goals, engaging in strategic planning, investing wisely, building resilience, and embracing continuous learning, you navigate the challenges and opportunities of the dental industry, ultimately building a thriving practice that leaves a lasting impact on your patients and community.

XI

Risk Management

1. Developing a Risk Management Plan

Guarding Your Fort: Building a Robust Risk Management Plan for Your Dental Startup

Imagine navigating your dental practice like sailing a ship. Strong winds – unexpected challenges – can arise at any moment. To weather these storms and ensure smooth sailing, a robust risk management plan is your essential anchor. This chapter guides you through building your plan, mitigating potential risks, and safeguarding the success of your startup.

Charting the Course: Identifying Potential Threats

Before setting sail, identify potential risks:

- **Clinical Risks**: Complications during procedures, adverse reactions to treatments, and other clinical situations.
- **Operational Risks**: Staff turnover, scheduling conflicts, technology failures, or equipment malfunctions.

Navigating by the Rules: Regulatory and Compliance Risks

Staying informed about industry regulations and compliance requirements is crucial. This includes:

- Changes in healthcare laws: Licensure regulations, infection control protocols, and data privacy guidelines.
- Implementing compliance measures: Regular staff training, adhering to protocols, and maintaining certifications.

Weathering Financial Storms: Managing Debt and Insurance

Financial risks can threaten your stability. Be proactive by:

- Managing debt: Develop strategies to minimize debt and have contingency plans for economic downturns.
- Insurance coverage: Secure malpractice insurance, business liability insurance, and coverage for unforeseen events.

Protecting Your Treasure: Cybersecurity and Data Protection

Patient information is precious cargo. Safeguard it with:

- **Robust cybersecurity measures**: Secure electronic health records, use encryption, and regularly update security protocols.
- **Staff training**: Educate your team on cybersecurity best practices and secure procedures.

Be Ready for Anything: Emergency Preparedness

Develop protocols for unexpected events:

- Emergency plans: Evacuation plans, emergency medical kits, and staff training for various scenarios.
- Communication strategies: Clearly define responsibilities, establish communication channels, and ensure everyone knows emergency procedures.

Crew Training: Investing in Staff Knowledge and Awareness

Empower your team to manage risks effectively:

- **Risk awareness training**: Educate staff on potential risks associated with their roles and responsibilities.
- **Continued professional development**: Ensure your team stays informed about evolving standards and risk management best practices.

Open Communication and Informed Consent: Building Trust with Patients

Clear communication is vital for informed decisions:

- **Transparent communication**: Discuss potential risks associated with treatments and ensure patients understand all options.

- **Informed consent**: Provide comprehensive information and obtain written consent documenting patient understanding and agreement.

Calming Choppy Waters: Conflict Resolution and Patient Complaints

Develop protocols for addressing disagreements:

- **Conflict resolution protocols**: Establish a structured process for resolving disputes professionally and efficiently.
- **Patient complaint procedures**: Respond promptly to concerns, investigate issues thoroughly, and take corrective actions.

Constant Vigilance: Monitoring and Evaluation

Don't let your guard down:

- **Regular risk assessments**: Identify new or evolving risks through systematic evaluations.
- **Performance reviews**: Assess adherence to risk management protocols and provide constructive feedback for improvement.

Keeping a Logbook: Documentation and Record-Keeping

Detailed records are essential for continuous improvement:

- **Thorough documentation**: Maintain documentation of protocols, training records, and actions taken in response to identified risks.
- **Incident report review**: Analyze root causes, implement preventive measures, and integrate lessons learned into your plan.

Building a robust risk management plan is not just about weathering storms; it's about building a safer, more resilient dental practice. By proactively identifying and mitigating risks, prioritizing compliance, protecting data, preparing for emergencies, investing in staff knowledge, fostering patient trust, and continuously monitoring and evaluating your strategies, you ensure smooth sailing on the journey to long-term success. Remember, your risk management plan is your anchor, keeping you navigating confidently towards a bright future for your dental practice and your patients.

2. Ensuring HIPAA Compliance

In the realm of dentistry, safeguarding patient information isn't just a box to check – it's the cornerstone of trust. The Health Insurance Portability and Accountability Act (HIPAA) sets the standards for protecting that information, and navigating its complexities can feel daunting. Fear not! This chapter serves as your compass, demystifying HIPAA compliance and empowering you to build a practice where security and transparency reign supreme.

The Heart of HIPAA: Protecting Privacy and Building Trust

Remember, HIPAA isn't just about avoiding fines. It's about protecting the fundamental right of your patients to privacy. Their health information is deeply personal, and ensuring its security builds trust and strengthens your reputation. Think of it as the foundation upon which your practice thrives.

Demystifying the Rules: Privacy and Security

HIPAA has two key components: the **Privacy Rule** and the **Security Rule**. The Privacy Rule dictates how you use and disclose patient information, while the Security Rule focuses on the technical and physical safeguards needed to protect electronic information (ePHI). Both are crucial for compliance.

Building Your Compliance Fortress: Safeguards and Procedures

Think of safeguards as layers of protection for your patient information. Here's how to build yours:

- **Administrative**: Designate a privacy officer, train your team, and establish clear policies and procedures for handling PHI.
- **Technical**: Implement access controls, encryption, and regular security assessments to shield ePHI.
- **Physical**: Securely store paper records, control access to devices containing PHI, and have disposal protocols for electronic media.

Consent: Empowering Your Patients

Informed consent is a cornerstone of HIPAA. Use clear and comprehensive consent forms to explain how you'll use and disclose their information. Remember, authorization is needed for sensitive disclosures like marketing or research.

When Things Go Wrong: Responding to Breaches

Breaches happen, but how you respond matters. Create a detailed incident response plan to address breaches promptly, notify affected individuals and authorities, and minimize damage. Regular security audits help identify vulnerabilities before they become breaches.

Working Together: Business Associate Agreements

When other entities handle your patient information (e.g., billing services), ensure their compliance with HIPAA through business associate agreements. They outline responsibilities and expectations, making everyone accountable for privacy.

Continuous Improvement: Training and Audits

Compliance isn't a one-time event. Regularly train your staff on HIPAA, keeping them updated on regulations and reinforcing safe practices. Internal audits help identify and address any gaps in compliance.

Staying Ahead of the Curve: Updates and Resources

HIPAA evolves, so stay informed! Regularly check for updates from the Department of Health and Human Services (HHS) and consider engaging HIPAA consultants for expert guidance.

HIPAA compliance isn't just about checklists and regulations – it's about building a practice where patients feel their information is safe and their trust is valued. By following these steps, you create a secure environment, navigate compliance with confidence, and ultimately build a stronger, more respected dental practice. Remember, patient trust is your most valuable asset – protect it fiercely.

3. Addressing Malpractice Insurance and Legal Protections

Like any good castle, yours needs strong defenses to withstand potential legal challenges. This chapter equips you with the knowledge and tools to build impenetrable walls, secure your assets, and protect your reputation through malpractice insurance and legal preparedness.

The Shield of Malpractice Insurance:

Think of malpractice insurance as your first line of defense. It provides crucial financial protection against claims alleging negligence or errors in patient care.

- **Understanding Types of Coverage**: Explore options like occurrence-based and claims-made policies, ensuring your needs are met. Don't forget defense costs and additional expenses.
- **Finding the Right Fit**: Research providers, compare coverage options, and prioritize those experienced in serving dentists. Remember, tailored coverage is key.

Lowering the Drawbridge: Risk Mitigation Strategies:

Proactive measures can make legal challenges less likely:

- **Communication is Key**: Establish clear communication with patients. Discuss treatment plans, risks, and expected outcomes transparently.
- **Document Like a Scribe**: Maintain thorough and accurate records of patient interactions and treatment plans. These serve as valuable evidence in legal battles.

Fortifying the Walls: Additional Legal Protections:
Your castle needs more than just insurance:

- **Incorporate for Protection**: Explore legal structures like Professional Corporations (PCs) or Limited Liability Companies (LLCs) to shield personal assets.
- **Know Your Domain**: Stay informed about state-specific laws and regulations governing dental practices. Compliance is your moat, keeping legal troubles at bay.

Facing the Siege: Responding to Legal Challenges:
Should legal challenges arise, be prepared:

- **Seek Wise Counsel**: Engage experienced legal professionals specializing in healthcare law. Their expertise is your strongest weapon.
- **Promptly Inform Your Insurer**: Report incidents and claims immediately to your malpractice insurance provider. Time is of the essence.

Sharpening Your Skills: Continuing Legal Education:

Never stop learning:

- **Stay Informed**: Participate in legal education programs specific to dentistry. Adapt to changing laws and risk management strategies.
- **Network with Experts**: Build relationships with healthcare law professionals. Their insights can be invaluable when navigating legal complexities.

Scouting the Territory: Risk Assessment and Mitigation:

Be proactive, not reactive:

- **Conduct Regular Risk Assessments**: Identify potential risks in patient care, documentation, and operations. Mitigate them before they become threats.
- **Train Your Troops**: Provide ongoing legal compliance and risk management training to your staff. Knowledge is power in your defense.

Keeping the Peace: Patient Satisfaction and Conflict Resolution:

Happy patients are less likely to sue:

- **Prioritize Satisfaction**: Deliver high-quality care and foster positive patient relationships. Prevention is better than cure.
- **Establish Conflict Resolution Protocols**: Implement clear processes for addressing patient concerns and disputes. Amicable resolution benefits everyone.

Maintaining Your Defenses: Reviewing Protections and Insurance:

Don't let your guard down:

- **Review Legal Structures Regularly**: Assess if your legal framework needs adjustments to keep pace with your evolving practice.
- **Annually Review Insurance Coverage**: Ensure your malpractice insurance remains adequate, reflecting changes in your practice and coverage needs.

By understanding malpractice insurance, choosing the right coverage, implementing risk mitigation strategies, incorporating legal structures, responding effectively to challenges, engaging in continuous learning, conducting regular risk assessments, prioritizing patient satisfaction, and reviewing your protections, you build a formidable defense for your dental practice. This chapter empowers you to navigate the complexities of legal matters, ensuring your practice thrives with both financial security and a strong reputation. Remember, a safe and secure castle attracts patients and fosters professional success. Build yours wisely.

XII

Opening Day Preparation

1. Finalizing Setup and Equipment

Orchestrating Your Dental Practice's Grand Opening

Your big day, opening day, is the culmination of months of planning and preparation. This chapter guides you through the final crescendo, ensuring your practice debuts with flawless execution and sets the stage for a successful future.

The Final Dress Rehearsal: Facility Readiness

Picture yourself as the conductor, meticulously checking every detail. Conduct a walkthrough inspection, ensuring construction is complete, adheres to regulations, and provides a safe and inviting environment. Test all systems, plumbing, electricity, HVAC – even water lines and suction! Address any glitches promptly to avoid opening day hiccups.

Tuning the Instruments: Equipment Calibration and Testing

Dental chairs, like finely tuned instruments, need to be perfect. Calibrate and test each operatory, ensuring comfort for both you and your patients. Verify lighting, controls, and equipment function flawlessly. Don't forget the diagnostic tools – X-rays, cameras, scanners – calibrate and test for accurate, high-quality imaging.

Maintaining Harmony: Sterilization and Infection Control

Sterilization is the silent hero of any healthcare setting. Verify your autoclave and other equipment function flawlessly, meeting industry standards. Implement protocols for routine maintenance and monitoring. Ensure you have ample infection control supplies, like gloves, masks, and disinfectants, and that proper waste disposal procedures are in place.

Preparing for the Unexpected: Emergency Preparedness

Emergencies can disrupt even the best-laid plans. Be ready with emergency kits containing essential supplies and medications. Train your staff on evacuation procedures and first aid. Display contact information prominently. Test communication systems – phones, intercoms – to ensure smooth coordination during emergencies.

Digitizing the Score: IT and Software Systems

Your practice management software is the digital maestro. Verify flawless installation and configuration. Test appointment scheduling, patient registration, and billing functionalities. Don't forget secure data backup to protect patient records and critical information. Regularly test restoration processes to ensure your digital assets are safe and accessible.

Rehearsing the Performance: Staff Training and Orientation

Your staff are the performers bringing your vision to life. Conduct final training sessions to familiarize them with the setup, equipment, and operational procedures. Address any concerns and reinforce the importance of exceptional patient care. Simulate mock patient scenarios to practice workflow and coordination, identifying potential bottlenecks and ensuring everyone is prepared for the real deal.

Playing by the Rules: Regulatory Compliance Check

Make sure you're hitting all the right notes with regulations. Verify that all licensing and credentialing requirements are met for both you and your staff. Review and reinforce HIPAA compliance protocols. Ensure everyone understands patient privacy practices and that safeguards protect sensitive information.

Inviting the Audience: Patient Communication and Marketing

Spread the word and connect with your audience! Confirm scheduled appointments and address any patient queries. Prepare a warm and welcoming environment with informative marketing collaterals like signage, brochures, and business cards.

Balancing the Books: Final Financial and Administrative Checks

Financial harmony is crucial for a sustainable performance. Test your point-of-sale systems for seamless transactions. Confirm credit card processing, receipt printing, and other financial components function correctly. Reinforce administrative protocols like check-in procedures, insurance verification, and patient record management. Train your staff to handle these tasks efficiently and with a patient-centric approach.

The Grand Finale: Team Motivation and Readiness

A motivated team delivers a stellar performance. Organize team-building activities to boost morale and foster collaboration. Conduct a pre-opening pep talk, emphasizing the significance of their roles and their contribution to patient care and practice success.

Opening day is not just about opening doors. It's the culmination of dedication, preparation, and a commitment to excellence. By following these steps, you ensure your practice launches with a flawless performance, ready to deliver a symphony of smiles for your patients and solidify your success in the years to come. Remember, the performance never truly ends – keep refining, keep rehearsing, and keep striving to create a harmonious dental experience for everyone.

2. Staff Training and Readiness

A dental practice isn't just about bricks and mortar – it's about the skilled hands and caring hearts that bring it to life. Your staff are the orchestra, and their seamless performance on opening day determines the symphony of smiles you deliver to your patients. This chapter guides you through crafting a training program that fosters not just individual competence, but a unified team spirit, ready to hit the ground running.

Setting the Stage: Facility Orientation and Equipment Familiarity

Start with a grand tour! Conduct a comprehensive walkthrough of your dental facility, introducing them to the layout, key areas, and emergency exits. Familiarization breeds confidence, so let them explore and ask questions.

Next, dive into the instruments. Provide hands-on training on all dental equipment, from chairs and diagnostic tools to sterilization systems. Ensure each team member feels comfortable and understands the functionality of their tools.

Mastering Their Parts: Role-Specific Training

Each member plays a crucial role in the orchestra. Train front desk staff on check-in procedures, appointment scheduling, insurance verification, and financial transactions. Emphasize empathy and clear communication – they're the first impression!

Equip dental assistants with chairside expertise. Train them on instrument sterilization, patient preparation, and assisting the dentist during procedures. Efficiency and clear communication are key to a smooth performance.

For your hygienists, delve into oral hygiene procedures, patient education, and instrument usage. Emphasize preventive care and building rapport with patients – they're the oral health champions!

Facing the Unexpected: Emergency Response Training

Be prepared for the unforeseeable. Conduct regular emergency drills to ensure everyone knows evacuation procedures, first aid protocols, and how to handle unexpected situations. Practice makes perfect, and calm, coordinated responses ensure everyone's safety.

Establish clear communication protocols during emergencies. Designate roles and responsibilities, emphasizing the importance of clear communication to ensure the safety of patients and staff.

Protecting the Melody: HIPAA and Patient Privacy Training

Every note must be confidential. Provide comprehensive HIPAA training to ensure staff understand the importance of patient privacy. Cover protected health information (PHI) handling and the significance of maintaining confidentiality.

Don't just tell, show! Use practical scenarios to illustrate applying HIPAA regulations in various situations. This hands-on approach allows staff to internalize privacy practices and apply them instinctively.

Harmonizing the Ensemble: Team Collaboration and Communication

A strong team isn't just a collection of individuals; it's a well-rehearsed ensemble. Facilitate team-building activities to foster collaboration and a positive work environment. Strong team dynamics mean efficient communication, mutual support, and a shared commitment to success.

Train everyone on effective communication strategies within the team. Emphasize clarity, respect, and active listening, especially in fast-paced situations or when dealing with patient inquiries.

The Power of Empathy: Patient-Centric Training

Make every patient feel like the star of the show. Prioritize customer service training to instill a patient-centric approach. This includes active listening, empathy, and effective communication to ensure patients feel valued and cared for.

Equip staff with strategies for addressing patient concerns and inquiries. Provide guidance on handling difficult situations with professionalism and empathy to maintain a positive patient experience.

Front Desk Finesse: Mastering Operations

The front desk sets the tone. Train staff on efficient appointment scheduling, considering factors like treatment duration, follow-up appointments, and the overall practice flow.

Insurance processing can be complex. Ensure staff are confident in verifying and processing claims, explaining coverage to patients, and addressing any billing inquiries.

The Encore: Continuous Learning and Development

The music never stops! Establish a culture of continuous learning and development. Encourage staff participation in relevant workshops, seminars, and training programs to stay updated on industry advancements and best practices.

Offer cross-training opportunities to expand skill sets. This enhances flexibility, allowing staff to support each other during peak periods or unforeseen circumstances.

Rehearsing for Perfection: Mock Patient Interactions

Practice makes perfect! Conduct simulation exercises to mimic various patient interactions, including scheduling, handling inquiries, and addressing concerns. This helps staff practice their roles in a controlled environment.

Provide constructive feedback after each simulation. Encourage them to share their experiences and insights, fostering a culture of continuous improvement and refining patient communication strategies.

Grand Finale: Motivation and Recognition

The opening day is the grand performance. Conduct a final pep talk to inspire confidence and motivate your team. Emphasize their collective contribution to the success of the practice and the positive impact they have on patient outcomes.

3. Ensuring a Smooth Patient Onboarding Process

The opening day of your dental practice isn't just about opening doors – it's about opening hearts and minds. That starts with welcoming new patients with a seamless onboarding experience that sets the tone for long-term satisfaction and loyalty. This chapter guides you through crafting a warm and efficient process, ensuring your patients feel cared for and informed from the moment they arrive.

Building a Welcoming Haven: The Reception Area

Imagine your waiting area as a prelude to a symphony – calming and inviting. Provide ample, comfortable seating that caters to individual and family needs. Clear signage guides patients effortlessly, while subtle background music and informative reading materials provide a soothing ambiance.

Streamlining the Journey: Efficient Check-In

First impressions matter. Implement a paperless check-in system using tablets or electronic forms, minimizing wait times and paperwork burden. Train your friendly and efficient front desk staff to warmly greet and assist patients, making them feel welcome and valued.

Empowering Knowledge: Patient Education and Communication

Informative brochures about your practice and services lay the groundwork for patient understanding. Introduce key members of the dental team with brief bios or visuals, fostering familiarity and trust. Consider having an educational video playlist running in the waiting area, engaging patients and promoting proactive oral health.

Transparency Builds Trust: Financial Discussions

Clarity is key to building trust. Ensure your fee structures are clear and readily available, readily discussing insurance coverage and out-of-pocket costs during onboarding. Designate a dedicated financial counselor to address patient inquiries and offer financing options, removing anxieties about affordability.

Setting the Stage for Comfort: Appointment Expectations

Prepare patients for their journey. Briefly explain the planned procedures, addressing any potential concerns. Communicate estimated appointment durations to manage expectations and anxieties. This transparency empowers patients to plan their schedules accordingly.

Soothing Nerves: Comfort Amenities and Distractions

Reduce pre-appointment jitters with thoughtful touches. Offer soothing background music, relaxing scents, or calming visuals. Provide engaging distractions like informative videos or engaging displays. These elements not only distract but also educate patients, fostering a positive association with your practice.

A Touch of Personalization: Welcome Kits and Care Instructions

Go beyond expectations with personalized welcome kits. Include essential practice information, a handwritten welcome letter, and tailored post-appointment care instructions. Consider adding sample oral care products to reinforce their role in maintaining good oral health.

Inclusivity Matters: Accessibility and Accommodations

Embrace diversity. Ensure your practice is accessible for all, featuring ramps, wider doorways, and accessible restrooms. Proactively inquire about special needs and adjust the onboarding process accordingly. This demonstrates your commitment to inclusivity and creates a welcoming environment for everyone.

Building Relationships: Post-Appointment Follow-Up

Show you care. Implement a feedback system to gather patient insights and identify areas for improvement. Thank patients for choosing your practice and expressing genuine interest in their experience. This personalized touch strengthens relationships and demonstrates responsiveness to feedback.

Continuous Refinement: Evaluation and Training Updates

Never stop evolving. Regularly review your onboarding process, incorporating staff and patient feedback to identify areas for enhancement. Update staff training based on these evaluations, ensuring everyone remains prepared to deliver an exceptional experience.

A smooth patient onboarding process is not just a one-time event – it's the foundation for lasting patient relationships. By prioritizing comfort, transparency, communication, and inclusivity, you create a welcoming and informative experience that fosters trust and sets the stage for long-term patient satisfaction. Remember, the symphony of smiles starts with the right first note – make it harmonious and memorable.

XIII

Systems Workflow Optimization

1. Implementing Effective Appointment Booking Systems

Welcome to the dynamic world of dental practice management, where the rhythm of appointments dictates the pulse of your daily operations. Effective appointment scheduling isn't merely about filling time slots; it's about orchestrating a symphony of patient care, provider efficiency, and financial viability. In this chapter, we delve into the art and science of appointment booking, exploring strategies to optimize scheduling efficiency while maintaining a balanced workflow that maximizes production and enhances the patient experience.

Understanding the Harmony: The Importance of Effective Appointment Booking:

Appointment scheduling serves as the backbone of your practice's operational efficiency and financial health. It sets the tempo for your day, ensuring a steady flow of patients while maximizing provider productivity and minimizing downtime. By mastering the art of scheduling, you create a harmonious environment that fosters patient satisfaction and practice success.

Diagnosing the Melody: Assessing Current Appointment Booking Practices:

Before fine-tuning your scheduling symphony, take stock of your current booking practices. Evaluate whether your scheduling strategy aligns with your practice goals and financial objectives. Are you maximizing production potential, or are scheduling inefficiencies hindering your practice's growth? By diagnosing these issues, you can tailor your scheduling approach to better meet the needs of both your practice and your patients.

Selecting the Right Instrument: Choosing the Ideal Appointment Booking Solution:

Explore the various appointment booking solutions available, considering factors such as patient preferences, practice size, and technological capabilities. Select a solution that integrates seamlessly with your practice management software and offers features like online booking, appointment reminders, and waitlist management. By investing in the right booking solution, you streamline the scheduling process and enhance the patient experience.

Conducting the Ensemble: Implementing the Appointment Booking System:

Ensure that your team is well-equipped to navigate the nuances of the new system, providing comprehensive training on scheduling protocols, software navigation, and patient communication. Communicate your systems to patients, offering clear instructions on how to book appointments through the new system and addressing any concerns or questions they may have. As the conductor of your practice, lead your team through the transition with confidence and clarity.

Composing a Masterpiece: Strategies for Efficient Appointment Scheduling:

- **Maintain Production in Mind**: Balance your daily schedule to ensure a mix of high-production and low-production procedures. Avoid scheduling a full day of low-production appointments, as this can lead to fatigue and diminished rewards at the end of the day. Train your staff to prioritize major procedures while filling gaps with lower production appointments to optimize daily production and maintain cash flow. Remember, you have bills to pay!
- **Balance Your Day**: Strategically plan your schedule to maintain a balance between high- and low-production procedures throughout the day. Avoid clustering similar procedures together, as this can lead to uneven production and inefficient use of provider time. Instead, stagger appointments to ensure a steady flow of patients and maximize provider productivity.
- **Seamless Double Booking**: When appropriate, consider implementing double booking to maximize provider efficiency. Train your staff to seamlessly manage multiple appointments simultaneously, ensuring that patients receive the attention and care they deserve. By strategically double booking appointments, you can optimize provider schedules without compromising patient satisfaction.

Appointment scheduling is the heartbeat of your dental practice, setting the rhythm for your daily operations and shaping the patient experience. By implementing effective appointment booking systems and strategies, you orchestrate a symphony of patient care, provider efficiency, and financial success. With careful planning, staff training, and a commitment to balance and efficiency, you can optimize your scheduling process to maximize production, enhance patient satisfaction, and drive practice growth. Let the melody of effective appointment scheduling resonate through your practice, guiding patients on a harmonious journey of care and creating experiences that leave a lasting impression.

2. Streamlining Patient Flow and Chairside Operations

In the intricate orchestration of a dental practice, the seamless flow of patients through each stage of their visit and the efficiency of chairside operations are paramount. Implementing streamlined protocols for treatments not only enhances patient satisfaction but also optimizes provider productivity and ensures consistent quality of care. In this section, we delve into the importance of establishing standardized protocols for various dental procedures and leveraging technology to streamline chairside operations for improved efficiency and patient outcomes.

Standardized Treatment Protocols:

Standardization is the cornerstone of efficiency and quality in dental practice. Establishing clear protocols for common procedures such as crowns, fillings, and extractions ensures consistency and reduces variability in outcomes.

For example, in the case of crown procedures, implementing a protocol where the dental assistant performs an initial intraoral scan upon seating the patient allows for immediate digital impressions. Following tooth preparation by the dentist, a focused rescan of the prepared tooth is conducted for precise digital modeling and fabrication of a temporary crown, minimizing chairside time and patient discomfort.

Similarly, for fillings, incorporating the use of a dry shield during treatment not only improves isolation and moisture control but also enhances the efficiency of the procedure by reducing the need for frequent pauses and adjustments. Standardizing the use of advanced isolation techniques ensures optimal conditions for restorative work and enhances clinical outcomes.

Leveraging Technology for Efficiency:

Intraoral scanners have revolutionized the dental workflow by enabling digital impressions that are faster, more accurate, and more comfortable for patients compared to traditional impression materials. Integrating intraoral scanners into treatment protocols accelerates the process of data capture, eliminates the need for physical impression materials, and facilitates seamless communication with dental laboratories for fabrication of restorations.

Additionally, the integration of chairside milling units heralds a new era in dental restoration procedures, facilitating the creation of same-day restorations that significantly reduce treatment time and bolster patient convenience. Through the utilization of CAD/CAM technology, dentists can seamlessly design, mill, and deliver custom restorations within a single visit, eliminating the inconvenience of temporary restorations and the need for multiple appointments. However, it's crucial to exercise prudent financial decision-making before investing in a milling system. While the allure of cutting-edge technology may be enticing, it's essential to conduct a thorough cost analysis to ensure that the investment aligns with the financial realities of your practice. Purchasing a milling system should not be driven solely by its novelty or market appeal; rather, it should be a calculated decision based on a comprehensive evaluation of the associated costs and benefits. In many cases, outsourcing scanning and fabrication to a dental laboratory may prove to be a more cost-effective alternative. Therefore, it's imperative to weigh the pros and cons carefully and make an informed choice that optimizes both clinical outcomes and practice profitability.

Utilizing digital radiography and imaging systems enhances diagnostic capabilities, improves treatment planning accuracy, and reduces radiation exposure for patients. Digital images can be quickly captured, analyzed, and shared with patients, facilitating informed decision-making and enhancing the overall patient experience.

Continuous Improvement and Adaptation:

As technology and best practices evolve, it is essential to continuously evaluate and update treatment protocols to incorporate advancements and optimize efficiency. Regular training and education sessions for dental team members ensure proficiency in the use of new technologies and adherence to updated protocols.

Soliciting feedback from both patients and staff members regarding their experiences with treatment protocols enables practices to identify areas for improvement and implement targeted interventions. By fostering a culture of continuous improvement and adaptation, dental practices can remain agile and responsive to changing patient needs and technological advancements.

Standardized treatment protocols and the integration of technology play a crucial role in streamlining patient flow and chairside operations within a dental practice. By implementing clear protocols for common procedures and leveraging advanced technologies such as intraoral scanners and chairside milling units, practices can enhance efficiency, improve clinical outcomes, and elevate the patient experience. With a commitment to continuous improvement and adaptation, dental practices can stay at the forefront of innovation and deliver exceptional care that meets the evolving needs of patients in today's rapidly changing healthcare landscape. Let the harmony of streamlined operations resonate through your practice, guiding patients on a journey of efficient and effective dental care.

3. Maximizing Productivity while Ensuring Quality Care

In the bustling environment of a dental office, striking a delicate balance between productivity and quality care is crucial for practice success and patient satisfaction. While efficiency is essential for meeting patient demand and optimizing practice revenue, it must never come at the expense of clinical excellence or patient well-being. In this chapter, we delve deeper into strategies and techniques for maximizing productivity while upholding the highest standards of quality care in a dental practice.

Leveraging Delegated Tasks:

Delegating certain tasks to skilled team members can significantly increase productivity while allowing dentists to focus on complex procedures and patient care. However, it's essential to maintain oversight to ensure quality standards are met.

For instance, temporary crown fabrication can be delegated to dental assistants, freeing up valuable time for dentists. However, dentists should oversee the process to ensure proper cleaning of the preparation site, accurate bite registration, and appropriate material selection to guarantee the longevity and integrity of the temporary restoration.

Additionally, cleaning the socket thoroughly after extractions is a critical aspect of post-operative care that should not be overlooked. Delegating this task to dental assistants under close supervision ensures that it is performed meticulously, reducing the risk of complications such as infection or delayed healing.

Optimizing Workflow Efficiency:

Streamlining workflows and eliminating inefficiencies are key strategies for maximizing productivity in a dental office. However, efficiency should never come at the expense of quality. Invest in reliable materials and equipment to ensure consistent treatment outcomes.

While it may be tempting to cut costs in certain areas, such as administrative tasks or office supplies, it's crucial not to compromise on the quality of materials used in patient care. Restorative materials, sealers, and cements are vital components of dental treatment and should not be compromised to save costs.

Laboratories play a crucial role in providing high-quality restorations and prosthetics. However, dentists must ensure that labs use proper materials and adhere to stringent quality standards. While digital scanning has led to cost deflation in laboratory dentistry, compromising on material quality can have detrimental effects on treatment outcomes and patient satisfaction.

Prioritizing Patient Communication and Education:

Effective communication and patient education are integral to delivering quality care and fostering positive patient experiences. Take the time to explain treatment options, risks, and benefits to patients in a clear and understandable manner.

While some aspects of patient communication may be delegated to dental assistants, dentists should remain actively involved in critical discussions, such as treatment planning and informed consent. Patients trust dentists to provide expert guidance and recommendations based on their individual needs and preferences.

Emphasize the importance of long-term oral health and the role of preventive care in maintaining optimal dental outcomes. Encourage patients to adhere to recommended recall schedules and home care routines to preserve the results of their dental treatment and prevent future problems.

Maximizing productivity while ensuring quality care is a delicate balancing act that requires careful consideration of various factors, including task delegation, workflow optimization, and patient communication. By leveraging delegated tasks effectively, optimizing workflow efficiency, and prioritizing patient communication and education, dental practices can achieve the optimal balance between productivity and quality care. Quality care is the foundation of long-term practice success and patient satisfaction, and it should never be compromised for the sake of efficiency or cost savings. Let the commitment to excellence resonate through your practice, guiding patients on a journey of optimal oral health and well-being.

XIV

Managing Dental Supplies and Inventory

1. Establishing Efficient Inventory Management Systems

Efficient management of dental supplies and inventory is not only essential for the smooth operation of a dental practice but also critical for ensuring high-quality patient care. A well-organized inventory system ensures that necessary materials are readily available, minimizing disruptions during patient appointments and optimizing treatment outcomes. Moreover, effective inventory management helps control costs, reduce waste, and streamline practice operations. In this chapter, we will explore in detail the steps involved in establishing and maintaining an efficient inventory management system in a dental office.

Establishing Efficient Inventory Management Systems:

To begin, conduct a comprehensive assessment of your current inventory. This involves analyzing existing stock levels, evaluating usage patterns, and identifying storage requirements. By categorizing supplies based on their frequency of use and importance to patient care, you can prioritize replenishment efforts and ensure that critical items are always available when needed.

Implementing a centralized inventory control system is crucial for streamlining management processes and ensuring accountability. Designate a specific area within the practice for inventory storage and appoint a responsible individual or team to oversee inventory management tasks. Develop clear protocols for ordering, receiving, and storing supplies, and establish standardized procedures for inventory tracking and documentation.

Utilize inventory management software or spreadsheets to maintain accurate records of stock levels, order history, and expiration dates. These tools enable real-time monitoring of inventory levels, facilitating timely decision-making regarding stock replenishment and preventing stock outs or overstocking. Regularly audit inventory to identify obsolete or slow-moving items, and dispose of expired or damaged products promptly.

Utilize just-in-time (JIT) inventory practices to minimize carrying costs and optimize storage space utilization. Rather than maintaining large stockpiles of inventory, order supplies as needed to meet immediate demand. Develop strong relationships with reliable suppliers who offer fast turnaround times and flexible ordering options, and leverage electronic ordering systems to streamline the procurement process.

Cultivate strong relationships with reputable suppliers to negotiate favorable terms and pricing agreements. Explore opportunities to collaborate with group purchasing organizations (GPOs) or dental supply networks to access discounted pricing and volume incentives. Monitor supplier performance regularly and hold vendors accountable for meeting contractual obligations, such as timely delivery and product quality.

Efficient management of dental supplies and inventory is a fundamental aspect of practice operations and patient care. By conducting thorough inventory assessments, implementing centralized inventory control systems, utilizing just-in-time inventory practices, and cultivating strong supplier relationships, dental practices can optimize inventory management processes and maintain optimal inventory levels. This commitment to efficiency not only enhances practice productivity and profitability but also ensures that patients receive the highest quality of care. Let this comprehensive strategy guide your practice towards operational excellence and continued success in delivering exceptional patient experiences.

2. Negotiating Supplier Contracts and Pricing

Negotiating supplier contracts and pricing is a critical aspect of managing dental supplies and inventory effectively. By securing favorable terms and pricing agreements with suppliers, dental practices can optimize their procurement processes, control costs, and ensure a reliable supply of high-quality materials. In this chapter, we will explore strategies for negotiating supplier contracts and pricing to benefit your dental practice.

Understanding the Importance of Negotiation:

Negotiating supplier contracts and pricing is not just about getting the lowest price; it's about establishing mutually beneficial relationships with suppliers that support the long-term success of your practice. Effective negotiation allows you to secure favorable terms, such as discounts, payment terms, and delivery schedules, while also ensuring quality and reliability in the products and services you receive.

Preparing for Negotiation:

Before entering into negotiations with suppliers, it's essential to conduct thorough research and preparation. This includes:

- **Understanding your practice's needs and priorities**: Identify the specific supplies and materials your practice requires, as well as your budgetary constraints and procurement preferences.
- **Researching suppliers**: Explore multiple suppliers to compare products, pricing, and service offerings. Look for suppliers that specialize in dental supplies and have a reputation for quality and reliability.
- **Analyzing market trends**: Stay informed about market trends and pricing benchmarks in the dental supply industry. This knowledge will help you assess the competitiveness of supplier offers and negotiate effectively.
- **Establishing negotiation goals:** Define clear objectives for the negotiation process, such as securing favorable pricing, establishing long-term contracts, or obtaining additional value-added services.

Negotiation Strategies:

During the negotiation process, employ the following strategies to maximize your bargaining power and achieve favorable outcomes:

- **Leverage competitive bids:** Request quotes from multiple suppliers and use competitive pricing to negotiate better terms and pricing agreements. Suppliers may be willing to offer discounts or incentives to win your business.

- **Emphasize long-term relationships**: Highlight your interest in establishing a mutually beneficial partnership with suppliers based on trust, reliability, and shared goals. Emphasize your commitment to loyalty and repeat business in exchange for favorable terms.
- **Bundle purchases**: Consolidate your purchasing volume and bundle orders to leverage economies of scale and negotiate lower prices. Suppliers may offer volume discounts or special pricing incentives for larger orders.
- **Negotiate payment terms**: Negotiate flexible payment terms that align with your practice's cash flow and financial requirements. Request extended payment terms, early payment discounts, or installment plans to improve cash flow management.
- **Explore value-added services:** In addition to pricing, consider negotiating value-added services such as free shipping, product training, or extended warranties. These extras can enhance the overall value proposition and justify higher prices.
- **Seek win-win solutions**: Approach negotiations with a collaborative mindset, seeking mutually beneficial solutions that meet the needs of both parties. Focus on building trust and fostering positive relationships with suppliers for long-term success.

Negotiating supplier contracts and pricing is a strategic process that requires careful preparation, effective communication, and skilled negotiation techniques. By understanding your practice's needs, researching suppliers, and employing proven negotiation strategies, you can secure favorable terms and pricing agreements that support the success and sustainability of your dental practice. Remember, negotiation is not just about getting the lowest price;

it's about establishing mutually beneficial relationships that create value for both parties involved. Let this chapter serve as a guide to navigating the negotiation process and optimizing your procurement practices for long-term success.

3. Minimizing Waste and Controlling Costs

In any dental practice, managing costs and minimizing waste are essential aspects of maintaining financial health and sustainability. By implementing effective strategies to control costs and reduce waste, dental practices can optimize their operational efficiency, improve profitability, and enhance overall practice management. In this chapter, we will explore practical methods for minimizing waste and controlling costs in a dental office.

Assessing Current Practices:

The first step in minimizing waste and controlling costs is to conduct a comprehensive assessment of current practices and procedures. This involves:

- **Identifying areas of inefficiency**: Evaluate all aspects of practice operations, from procurement and inventory management to treatment protocols and patient workflows. Identify any areas where waste is occurring or costs are unnecessarily high.
- **Analyzing expenditure patterns**: Review financial records and analyze spending patterns to identify areas of overspending or unnecessary expenses. Look for opportunities to reduce costs without compromising quality or patient care.

- **Engaging staff**: Involve staff members in the assessment process to gain insights into day-to-day operations and identify potential areas for improvement. Encourage open communication and collaboration to generate ideas for cost-saving initiatives.

Implementing Cost-Saving Measures:

Once areas of waste and inefficiency have been identified, implement targeted cost-saving measures to address them. This may include:

- **Streamlining procurement processes**: Consolidate purchasing activities and negotiate favorable pricing agreements with suppliers to reduce costs. Centralize the purchasing authority to prevent duplicate orders and minimize unnecessary expenditures.
- **Optimizing inventory management**: Implement inventory control systems to track stock levels, monitor usage patterns, and prevent overstocking or stockouts. Utilize just-in-time inventory practices to minimize carrying costs and reduce storage space requirements.
- **Implementing waste reduction initiatives**: Implement recycling programs for materials such as paper, plastics, and other recyclable waste generated in the practice. Minimize paper usage by transitioning to electronic record-keeping and communication systems.
- **Standardizing treatment protocols**: Develop standardized treatment protocols and clinical workflows to minimize variability in treatment outcomes and reduce unnecessary

expenditures on materials and resources. Train staff on these protocols to ensure consistent implementation.

- **Monitoring and analyzing expenses:** Regularly monitor financial performance and analyze expenditure trends to identify areas for further cost reduction. Set specific cost-saving targets and track progress towards achieving them over time.

Fostering a Culture of Cost Consciousness:

Creating a culture of cost consciousness among staff members is essential for sustaining cost-saving initiatives over the long term. Encourage staff to take ownership of cost-saving efforts and recognize their contributions to practice profitability. Provide ongoing education and training on cost-saving strategies and empower staff to identify and implement improvements in their areas of responsibility.

Minimizing waste and controlling costs are fundamental aspects of effective practice management in a dental office. By assessing current practices, implementing targeted cost-saving measures, and fostering a culture of cost consciousness, dental practices can optimize their operational efficiency, improve profitability, and ensure long-term financial sustainability. Let this chapter serve as a guide to identifying and implementing cost-saving initiatives that benefit your practice and enhance overall performance.

XV

Ongoing Education and Growth

1. Staying Informed about Industry Trends

The dental landscape is as dynamic as a healthy smile. To stay ahead of the curve and deliver exceptional care, lifelong learning isn't optional – it's the vital spark of your professional journey. This chapter empowers you to cultivate a growth mindset, navigate the evolving terrain of dentistry, and unlock the potential for continuous learning and success.

Cultivating a Growth Mindset:

Shift your perspective from "know-it-all" to "always-learning." Recognize that new discoveries and advancements happen daily, and staying informed paves the way for exceptional patient care. Embrace opportunities to expand your knowledge and skill set, and view challenges as stepping stones to growth.

Fueling Your Passion:

Professional Development: Commit to ongoing education. Explore diverse options like continuing education courses, workshops, conferences, and online programs. Actively seek knowledge that ignites your passion and aligns with your professional goals.

Joining the Tribe:

- **Professional Organizations**: Membership unlocks a treasure trove of benefits. Network with peers, access exclusive resources, and stay abreast of industry trends. Engaging with dental associations fosters a sense of community and shared expertise.

Immerse Yourself in Knowledge:

- **Industry Publications:** Subscribe to reputable journals and magazines. Delve into research articles, case studies, and technological advancements. Regularly absorb valuable insights from trusted sources.
- **Online Resources:** Don't underestimate the power of the internet. Follow blogs, newsletters, and online platforms focused on dentistry. These concise updates keep you at the forefront of emerging trends and best practices.

Embracing Digital Evolution:

-**Tech-Savvy Dentistry**: Stay informed about technology's impact on the field. Consider adopting advanced equipment like intraoral scanners, CAD/CAM systems, and tele-dentistry solutions. Embrace digital tools to enhance patient care, streamline workflows, and future-proof your practice.

Learning Beyond Borders:

- **Peer Collaboration**: Build connections with fellow dentists. Share experiences, discuss challenges, and learn from diverse perspectives. Collaborate on case studies and participate in online forums to broaden your horizons.
- **Mentorship**: Seek guidance from experienced practitioners. A mentor can share valuable insights, answer questions, and help you navigate the complexities of the field. Their wisdom paves the way for growth and keeps you informed about industry trends.

Investing in Your Team:

- **Staff Education:** Extend your commitment to learning to your entire team. Implement training programs to update staff on industry trends, patient communication techniques, and the use of new technologies. An informed and skilled team translates to enhanced patient care and practice success.

Staying Compliant:

- **Regulatory Awareness:** Be vigilant about changes in dental regulations, insurance policies, and compliance requirements. Regularly review updates from relevant bodies to ensure your practice operates ethically and aligns with current standards.
- **Compliance Training**: Proactively participate in compliance training programs. This ensures you understand and implement best practices, minimizing legal risks and promoting ethical operation.

Listening to Your Patients:

- **Patient Feedback**: Conduct satisfaction surveys to understand patient experiences. Analyze the responses to identify areas for improvement and tailor your approach based on their preferences.

Staying attuned to patient needs allows you to continuously refine your services and ensure they remain patient-centric.

Lifelong learning is not just an obligation – it's the key to unlocking your full potential as a dentist. By constantly seeking knowledge, engaging with peers and mentors, embracing technology, and actively listening to your patients, you transform yourself into a forward-thinking and patient-focused practitioner. As you navigate the ever-evolving landscape of dentistry, remember, the journey of learning is not a sprint, but a continuous smile-shaping adventure. Let this chapter guide you on your path to professional growth and excellence.

2. Participating in Continuing Education

The dental landscape is a tapestry woven with advancements, but without lifelong learning, you risk remaining a silent thread. This chapter unveils the power of continuous education, offering insights and strategies to fuel your professional growth throughout your career.

Redefining "Continuing Education": Beyond Requirements, Towards Evolution

Move past viewing continuing education as simply a box to tick. Embrace it as a catalyst for your evolution. By staying current with advancements, you elevate your clinical proficiency, expand your knowledge base, and ultimately, deliver exceptional patient-centered care.

Charting Your Course: Self-Assessment and Goal Setting

Before embarking, assess your strengths and areas for improvement in clinical skills, practice management, and patient rapport. This self-discovery empowers you to tailor your learning journey towards specific goals. Whether it's mastering a new procedure, implementing digital dentistry, or refining communication skills, setting clear objectives provides direction.

Expanding Your Educational Toolkit: Beyond the Traditional

While traditional in-person courses and workshops offer valuable hands-on experiences and networking opportunities, explore the diverse learning landscape. Online courses, webinars, and virtual platforms provide flexibility and access to content from anywhere. Remember, learning comes in many forms.

Deep Dives and Broad Horizons: Specialized Learning

Immerse yourself in advanced clinical training in areas that ignite your passion, whether it's implantology, endodontics, orthodontics, or emerging fields. Simultaneously, equip yourself with the tools to navigate the business side by attending practice management seminars and honing your leadership skills.

Pushing Boundaries: Advanced Degrees and Certifications

Consider pursuing advanced degrees or certifications to solidify your expertise and position yourself as a leader in your chosen field. Explore options like Master's programs in healthcare administration or dental management to complement your clinical prowess with powerful business acumen.

Building Your Support Network: Collaboration and Mentorship

Engage with professional organizations relevant to your areas of interest. Conferences, seminars, and networking events become gateways to connect with peers, mentors, and industry leaders. Remember, collaboration fosters the exchange of ideas and best practices, accelerating your growth.

From Knowledge to Practice: Bridging the Gap

Transform learning into tangible results. Integrate new techniques and procedures into your practice. This not only reinforces your understanding but also allows you to evaluate the practical impact of your acquired knowledge. Share your learnings with your team through training sessions, ensuring everyone is aligned with the latest advancements.

Technology: Your Learning Ally

Harness the power of e-learning platforms that offer a vast array of courses and resources. Explore immersive virtual reality and simulation technologies to refine your skills in safe, virtual environments. Remember, technology can be a powerful tool for personalized and engaging learning.

The Lifelong Cycle: Continuous Evaluation and Adaptation

Regularly evaluate and update your knowledge base. Refresher courses, revisiting foundational principles, and staying abreast of emerging trends ensure you remain at the forefront of your field. Remember, learning is a lifelong journey, not a one-time destination.

Leaving Your Mark: Sharing Your Wisdom

Consider giving back by becoming an educator or mentor. Teaching not only solidifies your own understanding but also empowers the next generation of dental professionals. Contribute to research projects or academic publications to expand the collective knowledge base of the profession.

Embrace continuous learning, and embark on a journey that transcends mere compliance. Become a dedicated and forward-thinking dental professional, leaving your mark on the evolving landscape of dentistry. This chapter serves as your guide, but remember, the true adventure lies in your dedication to lifelong growth.

3. Networking within the Dental Community

The dental community isn't just a collection of colleagues; it's a dynamic web of knowledge, support, and opportunity. Weaving yourself into this vibrant network goes beyond the transactional - it unlocks collaboration, fuels lifelong learning, and shapes your professional journey. This chapter guides you through exploring the value of dental networking and equips you with actionable strategies to build meaningful connections that enrich your career.

Embracing the Power of Community:

Beyond traditional associations, recognize the broader dental community. Peers, mentors, and experts become your collaborative village, fostering growth and enriching both your professional and personal life. Shared learning through diverse perspectives keeps you at the forefront of trends and equips you to tackle challenges together.

Leveraging Professional Societies:

Actively participate in dental associations and organizations. Find your niche, connect with colleagues, attend conferences, and stay informed. Consider contributing your expertise by joining committees or leadership roles. Not only does this enhance your visibility, but you become a force shaping the future of the profession.

Immersing Yourself in Events:

Regularly attend conferences and gatherings. These vibrant hubs offer unparalleled networking opportunities, industry updates, and discussions with thought leaders. Engage in interactive workshops and seminars for deeper dives into specific topics, fostering meaningful connections beyond large gatherings.

Building a Network of Peers:

Collaboration is key. Dive into case studies, research projects, or shared initiatives with fellow dentists. This deepens relationships and enriches the collective knowledge base. Attend social events hosted by dental associations - casual settings nurture connections beyond the clinical atmosphere.

Seeking Guidance and Sharing Wisdom:

Find a mentor, an experienced practitioner who becomes your guiding light. Gain invaluable insights and navigate challenges with their perspective. Don't forget the reciprocal nature of mentorship - offer your knowledge to those starting their journey, creating a symbiotic learning environment.

Embracing the Digital Landscape:

Establish a professional presence on platforms like LinkedIn. Actively participate in dental groups, share your knowledge, and engage in discussions. Explore virtual networking events or webinars, broadening your network beyond geographical boundaries.

Collaborating for Progress:

Engage in research collaborations or joint publications. Contributing to academic and professional literature not only strengthens relationships but propels the dental community forward. Share your expertise by participating in panel discussions or webinars, positioning yourself as a thought leader while connecting with diverse professionals.

Giving Back to Your Community:

Be a beacon for your local dental community. Host seminars, workshops, or participate in health events, enhancing your visibility while serving others. Join or initiate study clubs - smaller, focused groups for regular interaction, case discussions, and shared learning within your locality.

Partnering for Mutual Benefit:

Develop relationships with suppliers, manufacturers, and industry representatives. Gain insights into emerging technologies, access product demonstrations, and explore potential collaborations that benefit your practice. Attend sponsored events or exhibitions, actively engaging with both clinical and business professionals.

Weaving Threads of Connection:

Maintain consistent communication with your network. Share updates on your practice, achievements, and educational pursuits.

Regular interaction fosters long-term relationships and keeps you connected within the dental community. Support your colleagues during challenging times - a supportive network is built on mutual respect and assistance.

Remember, networking is a dynamic, reciprocal process. By embracing the power of community, engaging with diverse platforms, sharing your expertise, and offering support, you become an active participant in the shared success of the dental profession. This chapter serves as your guide to weaving meaningful connections, enriching your career journey, and making a lasting impact on the dental landscape.

XVI

Conclusion

1. Recap of Key Steps

Congratulations on reaching this pivotal moment in your journey towards practice ownership. As you stand on the cusp of realizing your dream, take a moment to reflect on the transformative steps you've taken thus far. This chapter serves as both a retrospective and a beacon, guiding you towards the next phase of your entrepreneurial adventure with renewed vigor and purpose.

Embracing Your Entrepreneurial Spirit

From the very inception of your career in dentistry, there has been a spark within you—a burning desire to make a difference in the lives of others. Now, as you step into the realm of entrepreneurship, it's time to harness that passion and drive. Embrace the entrepreneurial dentist within you, and let it guide you as you navigate the challenges and triumphs that lie ahead.

Empowerment for Our Generation

This guide was crafted with a singular purpose—to empower you, the aspiring dental graduate, with the knowledge and tools necessary to turn your dreams into reality. Armed with insights gleaned from seasoned professionals and industry experts, you are now equipped to embark on the exhilarating journey of practice ownership with confidence and determination.

Tailored Guidance for Your Journey

Recognizing that no two journeys are alike, this guide has provided tailored guidance to address the unique challenges and aspirations of dental graduates transitioning into entrepreneurship. Whether you're navigating legal complexities, honing your financial acumen, or crafting your brand identity, the strategies outlined here have been designed to resonate with your individual perspective and empower you to overcome any obstacle.

From Vision to Action: The Key Steps Revisited

Each step along the way—from self-exploration and goal-setting to financial planning and team building—has been integral to shaping your vision of a successful dental practice. Now, it's time to breathe life into that vision, to transform it from a mere idea into a tangible reality.

Charting Your Course with Confidence

As you chart your course forward, remember the foundational principles that have guided you thus far. Select your practice location with care, craft your brand identity with intention, and assemble a team that shares your passion and dedication to excellence. Embrace technology as a tool for efficiency and innovation, and master the art of sustainable financial management to ensure the long-term success of your practice.

The Power of Connection: Networking for Success

In the interconnected world of dentistry, the power of connection cannot be overstated. As you conclude this guide, take heed of the invaluable role that networking plays in your journey. Cultivate meaningful relationships within the dental community, seek out mentors who can offer guidance and support, and actively participate in events and initiatives that enrich both you and the profession as a whole.

Opening a dental practice is more than just a professional endeavor—it's a journey of personal growth, discovery, and fulfillment. As you embark on this exciting chapter of your life, remember to combine your clinical expertise with strategic planning, continuous learning, and a steadfast commitment to excellence. Let this guide serve as a roadmap as you navigate the twists and turns of entrepreneurship, and know that the best is yet to come. Here's to the realization of your dreams and the countless lives you will impact along the way.

2. The Startup Journey

The road to opening your dental practice unfurls before you, a tapestry woven with challenges, triumphs, and countless opportunities for growth. This chapter isn't just a source of encouragement; it's a compass guiding you through the exhilarating turns and exhilarating climbs of your entrepreneurial journey.

Celebrate the Dance of Challenges and Milestones:

Remember, challenges are inevitable companions on your startup adventure. Acknowledge them not as roadblocks, but as stepping stones that build resilience and sharpen your problem-solving skills. Each obstacle overcome becomes a testament to your dedication and entrepreneurial spirit. But don't forget to celebrate the small victories! From securing your first patient to completing the practice setup, take time to acknowledge and savor these milestones. These moments, big and small, fuel your journey and remind you of the progress you've made.

Embrace the Growth Mindset: Learning is Everlasting:

Foster a growth mindset that thrives on continuous learning and adaptation. The dental landscape is dynamic, and new technologies, techniques, and approaches emerge constantly. By staying open to these advancements and embracing a "learning is endless" philosophy, you position yourself for long-term success. Remember, every setback is not a failure, but a valuable lesson. View challenges as opportunities to refine your strategies, enhance your skills, and solidify your commitment to your vision.

Building Trust: Cultivating Patient-Centricity at its Core:

Your patients are the heart and soul of your practice. Nurture lasting relationships by fostering a patient-centric approach. Actively listen to their needs, prioritize their comfort and well-being, and deliver compassionate care at every step. Remember, word-of-mouth is your most powerful marketing tool. Exceptional patient care speaks volumes, attracting new patients and solidifying your reputation within the community.

Lean on Your Tribe: Finding Strength in Your Network:

The dental community isn't just a professional ecosystem; it's a support system waiting to be tapped into. When challenges arise, don't hesitate to lean on mentors and peers within the dental network. Their shared experiences and insights can offer valuable perspectives and encouragement. Remember, you're not alone in this journey. Cultivate a supportive team within your practice as well. A cohesive, motivated team contributes to the daily operations and creates a positive atmosphere that resonates with your patients.

Finding Balance: Harmonizing Work and Personal Well-being:

Building a successful dental practice demands commitment, but remember, maintaining a healthy work-life balance is equally crucial for sustained success. Prioritize your well-being by scheduling time for self-care, relaxation, and activities outside of work. Learn to delegate tasks and trust your team. Effective delegation not only reduces your workload but empowers your team and contributes to overall efficiency. A well-rested and balanced leader fosters a thriving practice environment.

Resilience: Your Superpower on the Startup Journey:

Challenges are inevitable, but remember, resilience is the cornerstone of entrepreneurial success. As you navigate hurdles, remember your ability to bounce back, adapt, and persevere will define the trajectory of your practice. Approach challenges with a growth mindset, seeking lessons and opportunities for improvement within each difficulty.

Passion as Your Guiding Star: Stay Enthused, Stay Inspired:

Never lose sight of your passion for dentistry. Your enthusiasm is contagious and plays a significant role in the success of your practice. Let your passion drive your commitment to providing exceptional patient care, advancing your skills, and continuously evolving your practice.

Looking Ahead with Optimism: Your Vision Is the Map:

As you begin your startup journey, take a moment to envision the future of your dental practice. Set clear goals, revisit your practice vision, and look ahead with unwavering optimism. Your dedication, passion, and entrepreneurial spirit pave the way for a rewarding and fulfilling career in dentistry. Embrace the adventure, learn from every experience, and remember, the impact you can have on your community's oral health is immeasurable. This startup journey is an exciting chapter in your professional story - own it, write it with passion, and may it be filled with growth, success, and the fulfillment of your vision!

Remember, you have the potential to be an exceptional leader in the dental field. This guide equips you with the knowledge and encouragement to navigate the exciting journey ahead. So, buckle up, embrace the challenges, celebrate the victories, and let your passion guide you as you build a thriving dental practice that makes a difference in the lives of your patients and your community. Best of luck!

3. Resources for Ongoing Support

As you set sail on the exciting yet uncharted waters of opening and managing your dental practice, remember, you're not alone.

This chapter serves as a navigational beacon, illuminating valuable resources and support systems to guide you through every stage of your journey.

Charting Your Course: Professional Associations and Societies

- **American Dental Association (ADA)**: This comprehensive resource offers membership benefits like continuing education, practice management tools, and a network of colleagues across the nation.
- **Local and State Dental Societies**: Engage with your local community of dentists for region-specific resources, events, and mentorship opportunities tailored to your unique landscape.

Lifelong Learning: Continuing Education

- **Dental Education Institutions**: Stay connected with dental schools and universities for workshops, courses, and programs to hone your clinical and business acumen.
- **Online Learning Platforms:** Explore convenient online platforms offering courses, webinars, and expert insights to keep you at the forefront of the latest advancements.

Finding Your Anchor: Mentorship Programs

- **Professional Mentorship Networks:** Seek guidance and practical wisdom from experienced practitioners through established mentorship programs within the dental community.

- **Local Business Mentorship Organizations**: Expand your perspective by connecting with mentors from diverse industries beyond dentistry, gaining valuable business insights.

Weathering Storms: Business and Management Consultants

- **Dental-Specific Consultants**: Leverage the expertise of consultants specializing in dental practice management for targeted guidance on operations, marketing, and financial strategies.
- **General Business Consultants**: Gain broader perspectives on business processes, financial planning, and leadership from general business consultants, complementing your dental expertise.

Connecting with the Ocean: Networking Events and Conferences

- **Dental Conferences**: Immerse yourself in the dynamic dental community at conferences, exchanging ideas, learning from industry leaders, and forging valuable connections.
- **Local Business Networking Events**: Expand your network beyond the dental sphere by attending local business events, fostering potential collaborations and fresh perspectives.

Keeping Your Compass True: Dental Publications and Journals

- **Dental Industry Publications:** Subscribe to industry publications and journals to stay informed about research, emerging technologies, and trends shaping the dental landscape.
- **Business and Entrepreneurship Magazines:** Gain broader business wisdom by reading publications on leadership, management, and overall business practices, applicable to your dental practice journey.

Sharing the Voyage: Online Forums and Communities

- **Professional Online Forums**: Join online communities where dentists share experiences, ask questions, and offer support, creating a virtual space for peer-to-peer learning and problem-solving.
- **Social Media Groups**: Engage with fellow dental professionals on platforms like LinkedIn and Facebook, exchanging knowledge, learning from success stories, and fostering a sense of community.

Harnessing Technology: Dental Management Software Providers

- Software Training and Support: Utilize training and support resources provided by your dental management software vendor to maximize its efficiency and streamline practice operations.

- User Communities: Connect with other users of your software through online communities, sharing tips, best practices, and troubleshooting advice to unlock its full potential.

Navigating Financial Currents: Professional Advisors

- **Financial Advisors:** Collaborate with financial advisors specializing in healthcare to ensure the financial health of your practice through strategic planning, investment advice, and risk management.
- **Legal Consultants:** Partner with legal professionals with expertise in healthcare law and dental practice regulations to navigate compliance and stay informed about changing regulations.

Finding Safe Harbor: Wellness and Support Programs

- **Professional Wellness Programs:** Invest in your well-being by exploring programs catering to the mental and emotional needs of healthcare professionals. Managing stress, maintaining work-life balance, and prioritizing self-care are crucial for your success.
- **Peer Support Groups**: Find solace and support in peer groups or wellness circles where fellow dentists share experiences and coping strategies, creating a safe space for open communication and shared understanding.

Embrace the collaborative spirit of the dental community, seeking guidance from seasoned experts and investing in your well-being along the way. While the journey may present its share of challenges, rest assured that with the right support, you possess the resilience and determination to navigate every obstacle that comes your way.

Your dedication, passion, and commitment to continuous learning are the guiding stars that will illuminate your path towards success. Approach this adventure with an open mind and a collaborative spirit, knowing that you have the resources and support needed to weather any storm and realize your entrepreneurial dreams.

As you set forth on this transformative journey, remember that the destination is not merely a thriving dental practice, but a legacy of impact and fulfillment that leaves a lasting impression on your community and beyond. With unwavering determination and the collective strength of your network, the possibilities are boundless. So, take the first step with confidence, knowing that your journey has only just begun, and the best is yet to come.

THE END

www.ingramcontent.com/pod-product-compliance
Ingram Content Group UK Ltd.
Pitfield, Milton Keynes, MK11 3LW, UK
UKHW021701190726
13853UKWH00001B/388

9 798869 197153